Palgrave Studies in Law, Neuroscience, and Human Behavior

Series Editors

Marc Jonathan Blitz
Law
Oklahoma City University School of Law
Oklahoma City, OK, USA

Jan Christoph Bublitz
Faculty of Law
University of Hamburg
Hamburg, Hamburg, Germany

Jane Campbell Moriarty
Duquesne University School of Law
Pittsburgh, PA, USA

Neuroscience is drawing increasing attention from lawyers, judges, and policy-makers because it both illuminates and questions the myriad assumptions that law makes about human thought and behavior. Additionally, the technologies used in neuroscience may provide lawyers with new forms of evidence that arguably require regulation. Thus, both the technology and applications of neuroscience involve serious questions implicating the fields of ethics, law, science, and policy. Simultaneously, developments in empirical psychology are shedding scientific light on the patterns of human thought and behavior that are implicated in the legal system. The Palgrave Series on Law, Neuroscience, and Human Behavior provides a platform for these emerging areas of scholarship.

Stephan Schleim

Mental Health and Enhancement

Substance Use and Its Social Implications

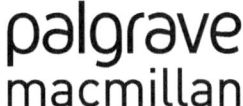

Stephan Schleim
Theory and History of Psychology
University of Groningen
Groningen, The Netherlands

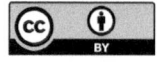

ISSN 2946-5192　　　　　　　　ISSN 2946-5206　(electronic)
Palgrave Studies in Law, Neuroscience, and Human Behavior
ISBN 978-3-031-32617-2　　　　ISBN 978-3-031-32618-9　(eBook)
https://doi.org/10.1007/978-3-031-32618-9

This Palgrave Macmillan imprint is published by the registered company Springer Nature Switzerland AG.
The registered company address is: Gewerbestrasse 11, 6330 Cham, Switzerland

DISCLAIMER

This book summarizes and discusses scientific research and is intended to neither encourage nor discourage any particular substance use. The use of drugs described herein may have negative effects on your health; their acquisition or possession may be against the law in your jurisdiction. Neither the author nor the publisher takes any responsibility or can be held liable for the consequences of any substance use or discontinued use as a result of reading this book.

*Towards a more consistent and rational way
to understand substance use.*

Foreword

Imagine that we could, when under pressure, just have a cognitive performance at our disposal that surpasses all of our normal possibilities. When we need it at peak time at work, in a private context to impress somebody, or to outperform others in a competition, it would be available for a limited time. Imagine that we could choose out of a selection of available, safe, and socially approved drugs. Moreover, we could time and manage its effects easily. Well, more realistically, such a performance enhancement would not be possible always. But even if it worked only sometimes—for a couple of critical situations in our lives—would this not be a nice possibility to have?

For precisely such applications, researchers have been looking for "cognitive enhancers". The drugs themselves would not solve our problems, but they'd help us doing so. They would empower us to make better use of our innate and acquired capabilities. It goes without saying that they should be safe and have as little side effects as possible. They should also be legally available and an interesting marketing opportunity for companies. Their effects would be so specific that they only improved our cognitive performance.

We are not talking about a wonder drug that could be applied for all purposes, that would guarantee eternal success and happiness. We also would have to be aware of possible long-term adverse effects or potential addiction that could come with the use of such "little helpers". We can imagine many possible scenarios that would seem enticing to a substantial number of people. Or would they, really? In the present book, we can find contemporary answers to many questions that arose with the search for effective "cognitive enhancers".

Stephan Schleim's book discusses how humans developed the idea of a pill that would help us to be better than we naturally are, in a domain that has increasingly been shaping who we are and what we achieve in life: our cognitive abilities. Related to our evolutionarily acquired ability to choose food also for its non-nutritional qualities, even animals can be observed to consume psychoactive substances. They seek and eat natural food that contains, for example, alcohol, because these animals learn and remember that a certain behavior can be performed much more efficiently with the drug. Such benefits can even make certain adverse effects, like a hangover, acceptable.

INSTRUMENTAL DRUG USE

Other researchers and I called this phenomenon "drug instrumentaliza-tion". This concept describes the use of a psychoactive substance beyond its immediate pharmacological effects on our emotional state. From this perspective, it becomes possible to understand why so many humans regu-larly consume drugs, even when they don't induce euphoria or an addic-tion. The substances simply are taken to facilitate other tasks.

Moreover, if already animals have a nervous system which allows them to learn and systematically retrieve such behaviors—drug use and its cog-nitive/behavioral effects—then we are likely to have this as well. As our brains are considered to be more efficient in many (though not all) aspects of survival, it is not surprising that our "drug instrumentalization" is more sophisticated than the animals'. Our repertoire of goal-directed behaviors is arguably bigger. Those involving cognitive problem-solving are cer-tainly the most diverse and complicated compared to the animal kingdom.

We also make use of a larger variety of substances than the animals can do. Our cultural history shows that we began doing so some ten thousand years ago. Originally, our human ancestors took drugs in their natural form and habitat: examples are cocaine by chewing coca leaves, alcohol by eating fermented fruits, and nicotine by inhaling the smoke of burned tobacco leaves. With the advancement of tool use, humans managed to improve their consumption habits. They then cultivated the respective plants to make their psychoactive ingredients available for a more system-atic use—eventually, up to an industrial production scale.

The last big advancement was to analyze the natural drugs and identify their psychoactive compounds. Advances in organic chemistry then allowed for a systematic modification of these chemical structures and thus the optimization of their neuropharmacological action. On the basis of this knowledge, also completely new compounds were (and still are) developed to facilitate cognitive/behavioral processes.

EMBEDDED IN CULTURE

Partially older than those industrial and pharmaceutical improvements, partially enabled by them, a rich cultural history of human psychoactive drug use developed. This is, by and large, not a history of "artificial paradises" where humans use substances to escape from a rather uncomfortable reality into the best of what our brains can produce in terms of euphoria and happiness. It is rather a sophisticated practice of use patterns that enable efficient drug instrumentalization.

In that way, different types of drugs were incorporated into "normal life" and to facilitate very specific jobs. There are substances to help us waking up (e.g., caffeine), to improve attention when it drops throughout the day (e.g., nicotine), to socialize with friends or approach potential partners (e.g., alcohol), or to relax better (e.g., cannabis), to name just a few examples. They support us in managing our complex lives with an ever-increasing demand for sophisticated behaviors, given that they are used in the right way and not excessively. In that respect, a drug that boosts our cognitive performance exemplifies just one out of many possibilities to make use of a psychoactive substance.

We can learn and maintain such behaviors. Now we only need to find more efficient drugs. One might think that, given our chemical ingenuity, efficacy, and safety testing, this should not be so problematic. Indeed, there are some successes: There are substances that allow us to concentrate longer when we get tired or to keep focusing on a cognitive problem when we become exhausted after a lot of work. Are they already the ideal "cognitive enhancers" some of us may dream of?

CHALLENGES

Well, all drugs that we know of come with numerous drawbacks. Firstly, think of their pharmacological profiles: They can be toxic at higher doses. They may also lead to tolerance development or even addiction. And, most importantly, so far no drug has been discovered or newly developed that would be truly capable to enhance the cognitive performance of a healthy, relaxed, and attentive human being. It really seems as if evolution did its best when shaping our neural networks.

Secondly, there are many social, ethical, and legal questions which need to be solved, even when we eventually find a safe and efficacious drug for this purpose: Should we really encourage its use and make it available for all? Or should we, at least in some contexts, even demand its use in order to maximize cognitive/behavioral performance? And what if that comes at the cost of a rebound effect after the productive peak? Would we really like to live in a world where our employers or peers ask us to optimize ourselves pharmacologically, as it occurred in professional sports when doping became a common phenomenon?

MENTAL HEALTH AND ENHANCEMENT

This book delves into the background of psychoactive substance use. In particular, this kind of human behavior is considered as a form of self-management of health problems, with a focus on mental health. Regaining and maintaining it is described as a common reason for using drugs. Stephan Schleim argues that mental disorders can best be understood as dynamic biopsychosocial processes, which continually change and may motivate varieties of substance use.

The consumption of prescription stimulants, particularly as the debates on "enhancement" or "brain doping" emerged, receives special attention. This book presents a highly entertaining and sometimes very surprising summary of this debate and its interaction with popular media. These media depend—often even financially—on the dissemination of breaking news, such as the (allegedly) rising numbers of students who were using these drugs to increase their cognitive performance. But Schleim's historical analysis illustrates that the current behavior is not a new phenomenon, before he discusses the best presently available evidence of such substance use in detail.

The book considers many other possible motives for drug use besides the frequently mentioned cognitive enhancement—and goes even beyond that by suggesting that what is often called "cognitive" might rather be reflecting emotional needs and coping with stress. This thorough analysis makes substance use understandable within a broader frame of drug instrumentalization. But the author also points out convincingly how difficult it really is when it comes to a clear distinction between the medical and non-medical use of a psychoactive drugs.

It goes without saying that there are also non-pharmacological strategies to improve the cognitive/behavioral performance that some want to enhance by taking a drug. These alternatives are discussed in an individual section. The author also addresses the problems of stigmatization and criminalization with their relations to present challenges for drug policy.

Schleim complements his timely and thorough discussion of the current debate and research with his personal conclusions about substance use. This will surely further stimulate the discussion. The author thus invites us to reflect on our own often highly integrated use of psychoactive substances for our daily activities and tasks. This setup provides an opportunity not only to learn more about oneself but also to put the drug instrumentalization theory to the test in real life.

Psychiatric University Hospital Erlangen   Christian P. Müller
Erlangen, Germany
March 2023

PREFACE

Just because alcohol is dangerous, indisputably, that doesn't mean that
cannabis is broccoli. Ok?
—Daniela Ludwig, then Federal Drugs Commissioner of Germany,
discussing the legalization of cannabis in the Federal Press
Conference of July 4, 2020

Early in the afternoon, I am standing in the newly built lecture hall which
my faculty, Behavioral and Social Sciences, regularly rents from the Faculty
of Science and Engineering to accommodate the high number of psychology students at the University of Groningen. It is the last lecture of my
course *Theory of Science* in which I emphasize the relevance of definitions
for research: why the way we classify the objects of investigation matters
particularly in the mind and life sciences.

As a teaser to get their full attention while their bodies are still digesting
lunch, I show them an advertisement from Germany, my country of origin, from the early 1950s. It focuses on women in everyday situations.
The first scene depicts a female customer standing at the counter in a deli-
catessen. She asks for capers, but the shop assistant apologizes, explaining
that they don't have any. The woman is getting angry, even furious: "What
kind of shop is this if you don't even have capers?", she shouts with indig-
nation. When she is about to lose her temper even more, the scene is interrupted by an animation. A bottle with the label *Frauengold* (German for
"women's gold") is floating on the screen while a calm male voice says:
"Don't get upset. Take *Frauengold*."

Then we see a second scene, now of two female employees in an office. One of them is upset about their boss, and her anger only increases while she tells her colleague how badly he treated her. She says that she is really "done" with this job, and grabs her belongings ready to go home, possibly even with the intention of quitting altogether. Her empathetic colleague cannot comfort her. Finally, the woman's anger turns into despair and she starts crying. Again, the scene is interrupted by the same animation. The voice repeats its suggestion to take *Frauengold* instead—but this time adds: "Then you will see the world objectively again." The advertisement ends with an illustration of what this "objectivity" looks like: The female employee now appears self-controlled, perhaps a bit ashamed, in any case docile, approaches her boss, an elderly man sitting at a desk in a dark suit, and apologizes for her earlier misbehavior. Everything seems well. *Frauengold* apparently does its job, helping women fit better into society.

There is another telling advertisement for the product, this time emphasizing a housewife's activities keeping the home clean and comforting her husband. This version plays with the promises of looking young and beautiful, having a fulfilling sex life, and an enjoyable time with the husband and children. All due to the work of *Frauengold*, the advertiser wants us to make believe. For reasons of time, I showed my students, mostly women around the age of 20, only the first version. They laughed at the woman getting so upset about capers. However, they then became silent and amazement seemed to take over. The social world they just saw on the screen must, I think, seem very different and remote. It is probably from the time of their grandparents or even great-grandparents.

I hope that the suggestion to solve social conflicts with a substance like *Frauengold*, containing alcohol and some herbs as the major ingredients, which was sold in Germany until the early 1980s, makes them think about our own lives. What are our challenges and conflicts? Might we also use substances to cope with such problems, that is, might we use substances *instrumentally*, to achieve certain aims and in a rationally understandable way? In between writing these lines, I just went to the pantry next to my office to get myself a cup of coffee which, an unwritten law seems to dictate in the Netherlands, must be freely available in all occupational settings at all times. To prevent students' unauthorized use of this service, an electronic payment system has just recently been installed. The standard amount deposited on my personal smart card is sufficient for 4000 cups— and refilled every day. "Free enough", one might think.

The *Frauengold* example has another advantage. It combines previous topics of my course, namely instrumental substance use, mental health, and enhancement, with the new and final topic: gender and gender roles. Although the advertisement does not present the product as a treatment for a mental disorder, it refers to coping with certain psychosocial conflicts and the mental processes that might arise in them, such as anger, impulsivity, despair, or anxiety. These are, in turn, associated with disorders increasingly diagnosed in our time, such as anxiety, mood, or attentional disorders. social phobia, major depressive disorder (MDD), or attention deficit hyperactivity disorder (ADHD) are more specific and, today, also commonly known terms.

Put together, these events inspire the working hypothesis under which this book is written: Firstly, we have seen a remarkably strong increase in both mental disorder diagnoses and psychopharmacological prescriptions over a few decades. Secondly, this is the period in which the debate on human enhancement emerged (or, as will be explored, reemerged), with most actors in the debate distinguishing strictly between treatment and enhancement. Thirdly, the boundary between mental disorders and normalcy is in itself fuzzy, and critiques of medicalizing more and more aspects of our lives—of excessively diagnosing disorders and prescribing drugs—keep being voiced. So what would happen if we looked at these trends from a different angle, namely that of instrumental substance use? Is there a *Frauengold* in our times? If so, which substance would it be? Painkillers, tranquilizers, antidepressants, cannabis, stimulants? Conceding that cannabis is not broccoli, are the regulations drawing significant distinctions between legal and illegal substances consistent? Finally, what can we learn about ourselves and the society we live in by understanding instrumental substance use and the aims it is done for?

Theory and History of Psychology,
University of Groningen, The Netherlands   Stephan Schleim

CONTENTS

LIST OF FIGURES

LIST OF BOXES

CHAPTER 1

Introduction

The celebrated list of 'human universals' compiled by the anthropologist Donald E. Brown includes 'mood- or consciousness-altering techniques and/or substances' as one of the essential components of human culture, along with music, conflict resolution, language and play. But there is little consensus regarding the origins of this universal impulse, which essential human traits it serves and how far back into our past its roots extend. Some have posited a primordial moment of discovery when proto-humans first encountered plants that expanded their minds to generate new forms of thought and language.
—Mike Jay, *British cultural historian (Jay, 2010, p. 10)*

Abstract This chapter explains the book's structure and also discusses the concept of health, how it is distinguished from disease on the one hand and enhancement on the other. While the definition of health of the World Health Organization from the 1940s is still popular, researchers recently developed a new concept which comprises six dimensions of human life; it also covers the active role of patients (self-management and adaptation) and the special interests of people living with chronic medical conditions, whose number keeps increasing.

Keywords Health • Enhancement • Normalcy • Mental disorders • Instrumental substance use

Three observations form the starting point for this book: Firstly, mental disorders are being diagnosed much more frequently, with psychopharmacological drugs increasingly prescribed as treatment. Secondly, cognitive enhancement or neuroenhancement is more often discussed in the academic literature and in the media. And thirdly, psychoactive substances—or "drugs"—are commonly being consumed for a variety of reasons. These topics will be addressed in turn: Chap. 2 focuses on mental health, Chap. 3 on enhancement, and Chap. 4 on substance use.

The link between these observations is the concept of *health*. Mental disorders are commonly diagnosed by a clinical expert when there is a cognitive, emotional, or behavioral problem associated with significant (1) subjective suffering and/or (2) impairment in one's daily activities. As an improvement beyond one's "normal" capabilities, enhancement is usually—and sometimes perhaps even axiomatically—distinguished from medical treatment. Lastly, whether a substance is perceived as either a medical or—a potentially illicit—"recreational", a "lifestyle", or a "smart" drug depends on whether medical and political institutions recognize it as a suitable treatment for a health problem. In 2003, the US President's Council on Bioethics contrasted treatment with enhancement in its report *Beyond Therapy: Biotechnology and the Pursuit of Happiness*, defining it as: "the directed use of biotechnical power to alter, by direct intervention, not disease processes but the 'normal' workings of the human body and psyche, to augment or improve their native capacities and performances" (President's Council on Bioethics, 2003, p. 13).

These experts—who included biologists, ethicists, philosophers, physicians, and scholars of law—were fully aware of the tentativeness of this distinction, as the quotation marks around the term "normal" indicate. Yet, for most of the bioethicists and neuroethicists, the latter being a new kind of specialist particularly addressing the ethical challenges of brain research, medical diagnosis mattered a good deal: They commonly discussed issues such as safety, coercion, or fairness related to the "nonmedical" use of performance-enhancing drugs, but barely problematized or even reflected on the sharp increase in the number of medical prescriptions. And that while the same substances were often consumed in both domains, medical and nonmedical—the majority, as we will see later, under a doctor's prescription. Physicians appeared to possess a magic wand: As soon as they declared something to be "medical", critical reflection became inappropriate.

Questions about, say, overdiagnosis or overprescription were left to medical sociology, which has traditionally investigated the process of *medicalization*. This term refers to extending the purview of medicine such that more and more problems of everyday life are first defined and then treated as *medical* problems (see, for example, Bell & Figert, 2012; Busfield, 2017; Conrad, 2005). Similarly, the complex field of drug policy was left to criminology, law, and addiction medicine, while many of the possible candidates for pharmacological cognitive enhancement are in fact strictly regulated substances—because of their "abuse potential", as the authorities say. This implies that people who take them are violating the law in many jurisdictions, literally becoming "illicit drug users", unless a physician has sanctioned their action (remember the magic wand).

The situation is made even more complex by the fact that the concept of *health* in itself—like "normal"—is ambiguous, with different accounts competing with each other. Since 1946, the famous and very broad definition from the preamble to the constitution of the World Health Organization (WHO) has defined it as "a state of complete physical, mental and social well-being and not merely the absence of disease or infirmity".[1] But if, for example, students' mental and social well-being significantly depended on them passing courses or even getting excellent grades, wouldn't that make their use of performance-enhancing drugs *medical*, whether they had a prescription or not? And, following this train of thought a bit further, doesn't social well-being also depend on the economy? Do we then need physicians to combat unemployment, inflation, or economic crises? This shows us how a broad definition like that of the WHO can turn virtually anything in our lives and societies into a medical problem.

More recently, an interdisciplinary team of researchers who featured on the title page of the *British Medical Journal* proposed that health be defined as "the ability to adapt and to self-manage" (Huber et al., 2011, p. 3). Doesn't that make the treatment-enhancement distinction collapse altogether? This is because the use of psychoactive substances to achieve particular aims in a certain social context could then be understood as successful adaptation and self-management. This argument can be reinforced still further by the "six pillars of health" that these experts validated in subsequent research, namely (1) bodily functions, (2) mental functions, (3) the spiritual/existential dimension, (4) quality of life, (5) social

---

[1] See the WHO constitution at: https://www.who.int/about/governance/constitution

participation, (6) and daily functioning (Huber et al., 2016). Health then ceases to be a distinct category and instead becomes a spectrum or continuum associated with virtually all aspects of our lives. Employing such a complex or holistic concept of health, all attempts to improve one's live with regard to any of these six dimensions could be understood as related to health and not specifically a kind of enhancement in the "beyond normal" sense.

The Aim of This Book

This book is intended as an *essay* in the literal sense, that is, an attempt to see what happens when the ever-problematic distinction between treatment and enhancement is abandoned. This effort is further supported by the fact that the domain of *mental* health is by no means clear, either: There, we witness the persistent absence of biological features (also called "biomarkers") to diagnose mental disorders in combination with often fuzzy diagnostic criteria and even "not otherwise specified" categories for atypical cases. This ultimately leaves it to the discretion of a clinical psychologist, psychiatrist, or other medical professional as to whether a person's psychological problem is deemed "clinically significant", as we will see in more detail in the next chapter. It is important to understand from the outset that the perspective taken here focuses on clinical experts and their institutions; it by no means denies the reality of people's problems, their suffering, or their impairment!

This book thus aims (or dares?) to ask what happens with cognitive or neuroenhancement on the one hand and a substantial proportion of the psychopharmacological treatment of mental disorders on the other if the treatment/enhancement distinction is set aside. How can we then make sense of the sharp rise in substance use over the past 30 years? Can we better understand this social change, this vast increase in the number of psychoactive substances consumed in many societies, if we investigate it more neutrally as *instrumental use*, that is, as individuals' decisions to achieve certain aims in personally or socially meaningful contexts? And are there any historical precursors that could guide our endeavor?

To answer these and related questions, we start with a deeper analysis of mental health and disorders in the next chapter. Philosophers have developed a useful framework to make sense of "things" that we will apply to better understand what these disorders, so frequently diagnosed nowadays, actually are. The concept of *addiction* will receive particular attention because of its close link to substance use. We will also discuss recent trends and scientific findings to evaluate whether the prevalence of mental disorders is actually on the rise, as media reports so frequently suggest.

From mental health in Chap. 2, we will move on to mental enhancement in Chap. 3, where we will first aim at a better understanding of the academic debate. A look at surveys on consumption will reveal how realistically leading scholars in the field and the media represent the (allegedly new and increasing) phenomenon. To do justice to the book's title and go beyond the scholarly discussion of neuroenhancement, we will also address nonpharmaceutical means to improve one's psychological functioning and mental well-being.

Understanding the essential basics of mental health and enhancement will allow us to look beyond these categories—and in particular the treatment/enhancement distinction. The focus of Chap. 4 will thus be *instrumental substance use*. It begins with a conceptual discussion of how we categorize different kinds of substances as "drugs" and what these classifications imply. The subsequent section on instrumental use will summarize several examples and answer the question of *what psychoactive substances are good for* when used properly. Historical examples will further support this way of thinking about substances. The subsequent section on moral values will describe different perspectives that we can take on that topic and thus provide guidance for drawing our own ethical conclusions. The fifth and final chapter will combine an overall conclusion with suggestions about further issues to investigate, and I will also draw a personal conclusion from my own point of view.

Mental Health and Enhancement: Substance Use and Its Social Implications thus combines knowledge and research from psychology and the social sciences, psychiatry and epidemiology, as well as philosophy and ethics. Present trends likely affecting hundreds of millions of people worldwide are put in a historical context (e.g., Jay, 2010), reflected upon theoretically, and contrasted with common frames in science communication. All chapters illustrate how concepts and definitions affect the work of clinical and scientific experts as well as the public at large, which in turn impacts on the concepts and experts' work. In doing so, the book will argue to avoid essentialistic fallacies underlying limited understandings of terms like "disorder", "enhancement", and "drug". Eschewing these limitations, *instrumental substance use* will turn out to be an alternative and more comprehensive analytical category to describe and make sense of people's behavior in various social contexts, which should also inform ongoing debates and decisions on drug policy.

References

Bell, S. E., & Figert, A. E. (2012). Medicalization and pharmaceuticalization at the intersections: Looking backward, sideways and forward. *Social Science & Medicine, 75*, 775–783.

Busfield, J. (2017). The concept of medicalisation reassessed. *Sociology of Health & Illness, 39*, 759–774.

Conrad, P. (2005). The shifting Engines of Medicalization. *Journal of Health and Social Behavior, 46*, 3–14.

Huber, M., Knottnerus, J. A., Green, L., Van Der Horst, H., Jadad, A. R., Kromhout, D., Leonard, B., Lorig, K., Loureiro, M. I., Schnabel, P., & Van der Meer, J. W. (2011). How should we define health? *BMJ, 343*, d4163.

Huber, M., van Vliet, M., Giezenberg, M., Winkens, B., Heerkens, Y., Dagnelie, P., & Knottnerus, J. (2016). Towards a 'patient-centred' operationalisation of the new dynamic concept of health: A mixed methods study. *BMJ Open, 6*, e010091.

Jay, M. (2010). *High society: The central role of mind-altering drugs in history, science and culture.* Park Street Press.

President's Council on Bioethics. (2003). *Beyond therapy: Biotechnology and the pursuit of happiness.* Dana Press.

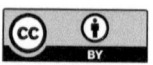

CHAPTER 2

Mental Health

Let us suppose [...] that the collective human spirit resembles a great
oyster. My goal is to extract the pearl. The pearl is reason itself, pure
sanity. I must therefore define the precise boundaries of what is
reasonable; anything else is madness, madness pure and simple. And
here is the definition. Sanity is the perfect equilibrium of all the
faculties, neither more, nor less.
—Joaquim Maria Machado de Assis *(1839–1908), famous Brazilian*
author (Machado de Assis, 1882/2013, p. 86)

Abstract This chapter introduces the notion of mental health as it is presently understood in the *Diagnostic and Statistical Manual of Mental Disorders* (*DSM*), which is published by the American Psychiatric Association. This is then discussed from the perspective of three philosophical stances, namely essentialism, social constructionism, and pragmatism. Historical examples—such as drapetomania, homosexuality, and schizophrenia—illustrate how culture, in particular thoughts about race, sexuality, and civil rights, can shape views on what is mentally normal and what not. Anticipating the later chapter on substance use, addiction receives special attention. Practical ways to assess dependence and also its definition in the *DSM* are introduced. Finally, the epidemiology of mental disorders is discussed. The question of whether the prevalence of these disorders is increasing is of special relevance. The chapter's interim conclusion is that mental disorders should be better understood as dynamic

© The Author(s) 2023   7
S. Schleim, *Mental Health and Enhancement*, Palgrave Studies in
Law, Neuroscience, and Human Behavior,
https://doi.org/10.1007/978-3-031-32618-9_2

biopsychosocial processes which can continually change; they are thus not concrete things (e.g., brain disorders).

Keywords DSM • Essentialism • Social constructionism • Addiction • Drug dependence • Mental disorders • Reification

The introductory quote is taken from the novella *The Alienist*, written by Machado de Assis toward the end of the nineteenth century. The "alienist" of the title, now an uncommon term, described the medical professionals who dealt with people's "alienation" from their (alleged) "true self". The term was later replaced by "psychiatrist", taken from the German language (Bynum, 1994). Machado de Assis's story is about a physician and scientist who, after being educated at the leading universities of Portugal and Spain, returns to his home country of Brazil to investigate mental health. The doctor's first attempt to distinguish sanity from madness is to define the former as the perfect equilibrium of all (mental) faculties. However, when he finds out that this means placing four-fifths of the local population in a mental asylum, the alienist revises his view. As a true scientist who applies statistical methods, he calculates that a disequilibrium of the mental faculties must instead be normal. This then becomes the new definition of sanity. Accordingly, the people in the asylum are released to make beds available for the remaining fifth of the local population (Machado de Assis, 1882/2013).

Although this is a fictitious example from a different time and culture, the question of *what constitutes mental health and mental disorders* is still important 140 years later. The answer is essential for our subject, as a deviation from the norm can be seen as justifying a clinical diagnosis, followed by psychological/psychiatric therapy and, often, psychopharmacological treatment. Defining "mental health" is as complex as defining what constitutes "normalcy", or "mind", or the subject matter of psychology and psychiatry. Fortunately, however, this does not make the answers completely arbitrary. In this chapter, we will learn about a few viable options. For example, the researchers who proposed the new definition of health and identified its "six pillars", mentioned in the introduction, have further deconstructed the pillar of "mental functions & perception" into cognitive functioning, emotional state, esteem/self-respect, feeling in charge/manageability, self-management, understanding one's situation/comprehensibility, and resilience (Huber et al., 2016). Their approach broadens the perspective for further research and policy on health.

The *DSM*

For actual clinical practice in psychology and psychiatry, it is more useful to have a look at the *Diagnostic and Statistical Manual of Mental Disorders* (*DSM*), edited by the American Psychiatric Association (APA). Its most recent version, the *DSM-5-TR* (APA, 2022), was published in March 2022. This handbook is best known for its hundreds of classifications of mental disorders in terms of checklists, some of which we will analyze in more detail below. It is less known for its tentative definition of what a mental disorder is, which we will discuss shortly. But first, it helps to know something of the manual's history.

During the two world wars of the twentieth century, the psychological assessment of soldiers proved to be a useful means of predicting the jobs and situations in which the servicemen would function well. An important aspect of this was mental health. In this tradition, the APA decided to develop a diagnostic manual for their domain (i.e., psychiatry), which was published in 1952 as the *DSM-I*. This edition and the second one of 1968 reflected the then prevailing Freudian view of mental disorders, including assumptions about their causes: primarily parent–child conflicts. Throughout the 1970s, however, psychiatric researchers became increasingly dissatisfied with this model. They wanted to develop a scientific version of the manual, eliminating speculation and increasing the inter-rater reliability, that is, the likelihood that any two clinicians would give a patient the same diagnosis (see Shorter, 2015).

A historical role model for this endeavor was the German psychiatrist Emil Kraepelin (1856–1926), who had distinguished only two mental disorders—precursors of what we now call major depressive disorder and schizophrenia—and tried to explain these in terms of brain damage. Psychiatrists in the 1970s hoped that breakthroughs in genetics and the newly emerging field of neuroscience would eventually allow them to objectify diagnosis in their domain. To meet the advocated scientific standards, the *DSM-III* that was published in 1980 no longer contained a causal theory (*etiology*, in technical terms), but only the symptom checklists that we still have today. These are complemented by information on the characteristics and prevalence for each category.

The Official Account

It is important to realize that this situation remained unchanged in the subsequent editions, including the most recent *DSM-5-TR* of 2022. This means that while a good deal of information has been gathered about risk factors, we still do not know in a strict sense what the causes of mental disorders are. This makes some psychiatrists worry that their field might be taken less seriously than other domains of medicine where there is greater knowledge of the causes of diseases available, as well as biological and—in this sense less subjective—diagnostic tools (Kendler, 2016). If we bear this in mind, we will better understand the tentative and pragmatic nature of the APA's official account as to what constitutes mental disorders:

> A *mental disorder* is a syndrome characterized by clinically significant disturbance in an individual's cognition, emotion regulation, or behavior that reflects a dysfunction in the psychological, biological, or developmental processes underlying mental functioning. Mental disorders are usually associated with significant distress or disability in social, occupational, or other important activities. An expectable or culturally approved response to a common stressor or loss, such as the death of a loved one, is not a mental disorder. Socially deviant behavior (e.g., political, religious, or sexual) and conflicts that are primarily between the individual and society are not mental disorders [...]. (APA, 2022)[1]

The authors concede that this is only an approximation. Nevertheless, taking a closer look at this working definition will tell us a lot about mental health: Firstly, it is important to understand that there is no objective standard for "clinical significance". It is ultimately up to the clinical experts to assess the severity of a person's problems—and particularly whether they deserve or even require professional help, for which a diagnosis is then given. Secondly, the subsequent listing of cognition, emotion and behavior on the one hand and psychology, biology, and development on the other can be said to describe the purview of psychology and psychiatry. It is true, again, that this is a pragmatic decision, and valid questions could be raised about the boundary with, say, neurology (Schleim, 2009). But we must presume *something* if we do not simply wish to engage in endless foundational discussions.

---

[1] I am quoting from the online version at https://dsm.psychiatryonline.org and cannot therefore provide page numbers.

Thirdly, suffering and/or impairment in everyday life are essential aspects of mental disorders. While the authors state that disorders are "usually associated" with these aspects, it is a rather philosophical question as to whether we can speak of the presence of a mental disorder if there is neither suffering nor impairment. Fourthly, the fact that "expectable or culturally approved responses" are exempted further emphasizes the normative nature of this definition. Note that "clinical significance" already expressed a norm (see also Stier, 2013; Tebartz van Elst, 2021). The fifth and last point requires that mental disorders are not primarily about a conflict between the individual and society. Why this is added so prominently here will become clearer when we discuss some historical examples later in this chapter.

Some readers may be surprised that the definition differs from what they have been told about mental disorders. Perhaps they believed that these disorders are medical diseases caused by a certain biological dysfunction, such as a biochemical imbalance in the brain, a genetic defect, or faulty neural circuits. That last notion was literally communicated to a broader audience several years ago by no less a person than Thomas Insel, at that time director of the US National Institute of Mental Health, probably the world's largest psychiatric research institution (Insel, 2010). His successor reinforced this idea a little later in a scientific publication and described the discipline as "circuit psychiatry" (Gordon, 2016).

It is thus important to understand that the definition that we discussed briefly above—which makes no reference at all to "circuits"—is not proposed by someone from, say, the anti-psychiatry movement. Instead, it is—and has been for decades—the official account of the American Psychiatric Association. When we learn about classic views to make sense of things in the next section, it will become clearer why experts can have such different understandings of mental disorders. The fact that the authors of the DSM actually called them "syndromes" further emphasizes the tentativeness of the definition.

2.1   THREE CLASSIC VIEWS TO MAKE SENSE OF THINGS

Science—as well as its predecessor natural philosophy, at least since Aristotle (384–322 BC)—has always attempted to categorize and classify things in the world, to develop *taxonomies*. Plants, for example, were distinguished according to their growth and flowering patterns, what they looked like (their *morphology*), and, more recently, on the basis of their genome. Likewise, animals were not always separated into categories such as vertebrates, which includes amphibians, birds, fish, mammals, and reptiles, but in earlier times they were separated according to whether they had fur or were furless, had blood or were bloodless, how many legs they had, and so on (Kendler, 2009). This exemplifies how people used what they knew and believed to make sense of the world around them.

The *DSM* is also a classification system, albeit for psychological problems. The categorization is intended to help clinical experts to understand and explain a patient's situation, to guide therapy, and to provide information about the prognosis. From a philosophical point of view, we can discuss three more general accounts to distinguish things, all with their own answers about how to build a classification system: *essentialism, social constructionism*, and *pragmatism*. We will learn about their meaning, benefits and limitations in this section.

Essentialism

Essentialism assumes that things have an intrinsic quality, an *essence*, to distinguish them. The standard model for this is the periodic table of the chemical elements, based on their atomic number (i.e., the number of protons). For example, something is iron if—and only if—it has 26 protons. It is not simply that atoms with so many protons are on average iron or that they sometimes have 24 (chromium) or 47 (silver). It is really quite straightforward: If an atom has precisely that number, it is iron; otherwise, it has to be something else. Note that this presumes philosophical *realism*, the view that there is an outside world that is independent of us conscious beings. It is not just by virtue of *our* counting and describing protons that something is iron and something else is not; this also implies that the chemical elements were like this before we started to investigate them scientifically, in fact even before any humans existed.

This straightforwardness is essentialism's huge advantage. If you want to find out what kind of thing something is, you simply look at its essence. As simple and clear as this might seem, it is also very limited. In the world of biology, for example, things quickly become so complex and variable that we lack a straightforward answer to the question of what constitutes their essences. Such cases also exist in the domain of inanimate physics: For example, it is both entertaining and educational to learn about the different attempts that physicists specializing in crystal structures have made to classify snowflakes.[2]

But why is this relevant to the classification of mental disorders? Around the year 1900, when Kraepelin's influence was at its peak, the discovery that progressive paralysis and other severe psychological symptoms—such as depression, mania, and psychoses—could be caused by infection with the bacterium *Treponema pallidum*, better known as the disease syphilis, had a huge impact on the medical world (Kendler et al., 2011). At last there was an example of how biological pathology could cause mental pathology! This also had major implications for patients. Thanks to the discovery of the antibacterial effects of penicillin a few decades later, the final and most severe stage of syphilis, with its disconcerting psychological symptoms, could be prevented. Although it is questionable to call the bacterium "the essence" of these problems, as the course of the disease differs between people and not every patient suffers the neurological damage associated with the psychological symptoms, the parallel with essentialism is obvious. For now, there were at least some clinical cases where psychiatric problems could be linked to an independent causal agent in the sense of realism and the general view of medical diseases, and this knowledge could even be utilized for therapy.

Thomas Insel reiterated this view when he informed the public at large that "faulty circuits" or "malfunctioning connections" underlie psychiatric disorders and that this knowledge is "forcing psychiatrists to rethink the causes of mental illness" (Insel, 2010, p. 44). He described area 25 in the brain as part of the "depression circuit". He also provided similar descriptions of the "faulty circuits" underlying attention-deficit hyperactivity disorder (ADHD), obsessive compulsive disorder (OCD), and post-traumatic stress disorder (PTSD). Insel compared treating depression by means of electrical stimulation of area 25 with "rebooting" a frozen computer. Those unfamiliar with neuroscience should know that the categorization of "area 25" itself stems from an outdated brain map—another classification system—which is more than 100 years old and does not meet present scientific standards (Zilles & Amunts, 2010). This and the knowledge that, as in the case of syphilis, psychological symptoms can be linked to

---

[2] See, for example, the "Guide to Snowflakes" developed by Kenneth G. Libbrecht, Professor of Physics at the California Institute of Technology, at https://www.its.caltech.edu/~atomic/snowcrystals/class/class-old.htm

these neural processes in some but not all cases, illustrate the hypothetical nature of this neurobiological model.

Another important fact is that none of the breakthroughs that Insel predicted for 2020, such as using brain scanners to diagnose mental disorders, were actually achieved. Meanwhile, other psychiatrists criticized the fact that their discipline's strong focus on the brain and nervous system hindered the further development or application of evidence-based therapeutic and preventive approaches (Lewis-Fernandez et al., 2016). They felt that the one-sidedness of the research agenda was harming patients. Yet Insel's position is just a simplified example of the influential view that mental disorders are brain disorders, closely associated with both essentialism and realism. But in the mid-nineteenth century, long before our time and even before Kraepelin, this view had been developed by another German psychiatrist, Wilhelm Griesinger (1817–1868), who is still sometimes referred to as the "father of neuropsychiatry". In 1845, he wrote in his then influential textbook on psychiatry:

> The first step towards a knowledge of the symptoms is their locality—to which organ do the indications of the disease belong? what organ must necessarily and invariably be diseased where there is madness? The answer to these questions is preliminary to all advancement in the study of mental disease. Physiological and pathological facts show us that this organ can only be the brain; we therefore primarily, and in every case of mental disease, recognise a morbid action of that organ. (Griesinger, 1845/1867, p. 1)

In line with this thinking, American psychiatrists (and not only they) set out in around 2000 to finally build a classification system guided by biology, combining data on genetic abnormalities, on "faulty circuits", and from neuroimaging—in short, "biomarkers" (Hyman, 2007; Kupfer et al., 2002). To put it differently, the *DSM-5*, eventually published in 2013, was intended as the first *DSM* to feature a true *pathophysiology* (literally: a physiology-based system of diseases). But if we now study the common and influential diagnostic manual of the APA, not a single reliable biomarker is reported in spite of the hundreds of mental disorders distinguished in it (Frisch, 2016; Schleim, 2022a). It is important to emphasize once again that this does not make people's psychological problems any less real. It shows instead—and we now have almost 200 years of evidence to support this—that the biological level associated with essentialism and realism does not provide an accurate account of mental disorders.

This does not require us, as is sometimes responded at that point of the argumentation, to assume the existence of an immaterial soul either. Instead, the present outcome is understandable when we realize the sheer diversity of people and their mental life and that even much simpler thoughts and emotions cannot be linked to unique neural signatures, also within psychology at large (see also Anderson et al., 2013; Schleim, 2022a). There is thus a good reason to have independent disciplines such as psychology and psychiatry alongside biology and neurology. The objects of investigation in the former fields are actually culturally formed and situationally embedded *subjects*—not atoms, molecules, or brain circuits (Hyman, 2021; Schleim, 2022b; Varela et al., 2017). This paves the way for an alternative view such as social constructionism.

Social Constructionism

Roughly halfway through the twentieth century, sociologists developed sophisticated views on how some knowledge is socially constructed, that is, brought into the world by us humans and our social institutions (Berger & Luckmann, 1966). Such discussions often go wrong when people misunderstand "socially constructed" to mean "less real". This may be due to an incomplete understanding of philosophical realism, which we briefly addressed in the previous section: the view that there is an observer-independent world, such as the chemical elements distinguished by their atomic number. Social constructionism obviously differs from realism in that it describes facts brought into being by human activities. The aversion of some to such social constructs may be understandable if we reflect on the common view that only natural sciences are "hard sciences" and that psychology, psychiatry, and the social sciences must therefore somehow be of a lower status unless backed up by "hard science".

The fact that evolutionary, biological, or neuropsychology as well as biological or neuropsychiatry have so many supporters is probably because these scientists are worried that their knowledge will not be taken seriously enough if it cannot be described in biological or neuroscientific terms (see, for an example, Kendler, 2016). It goes beyond the scope of this book but deserves at least mention here that the implications of quantum physics and its mathematical formalization for realism continue to be debated even a century after its breakthroughs. To put it differently, the "hardness" of the most basic physics known so far is not all that clear and some interpretations emphasize how the results of experimentation are produced by the human observers themselves (Faye, 2019; Gribbin, 1995).

The upshot of the previous section was that essentialism has failed for mental disorders at the classification level, particularly because there were remarkably few examples to support this view for almost 200 years. This is especially odd compared to the dominance that biological psychiatry has gained within research and treatment. Similarly, therapies based on the brain-based view of mental disorders have repeatedly provoked strong criticism, including within science itself. Telling examples are brain stimulation and neurosurgery in the 1950s to 1970s (Schleim, 2021; Valenstein, 1974) and—more recently and not for the first time—psychopharmacology (Hengartner, 2022; Margraf & Schneider, 2016; Moncrieff et al., 2022). These are complex issues that we cannot address here in detail, but fortunately we do not have to. For our purpose, it suffices to understand that the present situation calls for a different answer to the question of *what kind of things mental disorders are*. This will also pave the way for another perspective on mental enhancement and substance use in the later chapters.

Social constructionism emphasizes the importance of certain human actors and powerful institutions in drawing a line between what is considered normal and abnormal in the psychological domain. The psychiatrist in Machado de Assis's novella described at the beginning of this chapter is not only an individual in a power position but also a representative of medicine and science, both powerful social institutions. The fact that the doctor first put 80% of the local population into the mental asylum on the assumption that insanity is a disequilibrium of the psychological faculties and then, after finding out that this was at odds with the statistics, hospitalized only the other 20% under the opposite definition, is a fictitious and oversimplified yet telling example. Unfortunately, the implications of drawing this line are not always as funny as it may seem here, as we will shortly find out. *The Alienist* vividly illustrates the severe consequences that a mere definition by an authority, and as such a social construct, can have on the world and the people in it.

Excursion: What Is Money?

Before returning to our modern world of mental health, let us discuss a final example for those still committing the "less real" fallacy about social constructs. Open your wallet and take a look at a banknote or, alternatively, check your bank account. *What kind of thing is money?* I have European euros, US dollars, Swiss francs, and Indian rupees at my disposal. What all the notes have in common is the name of an institution or its representative (namely, Mario Draghi, former president of the European Central Bank, the US Federal Reserve, the Swiss National Bank, and the Reserve Bank of India). These institutions have been granted the privilege—established by law, another social institution—of issuing money in a certain currency. Anyone printing such notes without authorization will be prosecuted for forgery and severely punished. Until the Bretton Woods System ended in 1971, money had to be backed up by a certain amount of gold (about 0.89 gram per US dollar). As one of the basic elements (atomic number 79), this may be understood as an essence. The paper notes then simply were more convenient to use in daily life than heavy gold coins and bars.

That system was replaced by the present fiat currency model allowing central banks to create money at will. But private banks can also do this to a certain extent. Imagine having 1000 of your local currency in your bank account. This actually means that you are lending this amount to the bank until you withdraw or transfer it. Depending on the precise legal regulations, the bank can in turn lend, say, up to 9000 to other clients simply by putting that number on their account, expecting it to be returned at a later time and including interest. This whole system is based on the trust—a psychological process—that people can trade money for their desired goods and services and that loans will be settled.

Importantly, although money is a social construct that is literally created by central or private banks, thus human agents and institutions, much of our life deals with this "thing". For example, people work many hours to acquire it, some even risking their health or lives (think of police officers, sex workers, soldiers, or mercenaries). Fiat money in particular is not a physical thing. Even if you had a machine creating perfect copies of the paper notes atom by atom, you would still be prosecuted for forgery and the counterfeit notes would be destroyed. This foray into the nature of money illustrates that we may have good reason to overturn the "less real" fallacy. For our everyday lives at least, psychological processes and social constructs apparently matter much more and are in this sense "more real" than the entities that some natural scientists deal with by virtue of their profession.

Social Constructionism: Historical Examples

But what does this mean for mental disorders? Is their classification really as arbitrary as Machado de Assis's *The Alienist* suggested in the nineteenth century? Those arguing in favor of a constructionist view often refer to examples such as *drapetomania*, diagnoses of *schizophrenia* during the US civil rights movement, and *homosexuality*. The former two illustrate the abuse of psychiatry for racial discrimination purposes, the last for discrimination based on sexual preference. Let us discuss them here briefly.

To be fair to present-day psychiatry, the first example is not only very old and extreme but it also never became widely accepted in the medical domain. It is nevertheless an illustrative case of how wrong things can go when declaring certain psychological processes or behaviors to be pathological. On March 12, 1851, the American physician Samuel A. Cartwright (1793–1863) gave a speech on the "Disease and Physical Peculiarities of the Negro Race" at the annual meeting of the Medical Association of Louisiana, later also published in its journal (Cartwright, 1851). The doctor talked about "drapetomania, or the disease causing negroes to run away". The word is derived from the Greek term for a runaway slave (*drapetes*) and an old term for madness (*mania*).

Cartwright described the "disease" as "unknown to our medical authorities", but "its diagnostic symptom, the absconding from service" (ibid, p. 711), as well-known to overseers. In contrast to common accounts on the internet, this racist physician did not suggest whipping the slaves as a standard "treatment" for drapetomania. Instead, Cartwright described how it could successfully be prevented: by treating the slaves as neither too equal, nor too unequal. The captives should be held with some degree of comfort, but not too much, and with not too much brutality either. The doctor compared the "proper" relationship between master and slave to that between parent and child. Causes of the slaves' discontent should, where possible, be removed. Only when that did not work should punishment be used to force them into submission.

The (for us) incredible idea of framing a human being's desire for freedom as a disease or madness can be better understood when we realize that many whites at that time and place firmly believed that enslavement was the natural condition for blacks (see also Follett, 2005; Willoughby, 2018). Only a few years after Cartwright's lecture, many would fight (and actually lose or even die) in the American Civil War to uphold this order.

Within that racist framework, the doctor was convinced that he was performing a public service for the betterment of humankind. In a similar fashion, until the 1970s—thus 120 years after the proposal of drapetomania—psychologists and psychiatrists would perceive it as a public service to "instigate" heterosexual sexual behavior in people, particularly men, who had a sexual desire for people of their own gender. For example, David H. Barlow, who later held professorships in psychology at US universities and became president of the Division of Clinical Psychology of the American Psychological Association in 1993, concluded the following in a review article titled "Increasing heterosexual responsiveness in the treatment of sexual deviation" and published in the scientific journal *Behavior Therapy* in 1973:

> In view of the long-standing agreement among therapists on the importance of instigating heterosexual behavior, it is surprising how little research has been done. [...] Pairing procedures or fading techniques [...] are designed to instigate heterosexual arousal while social retraining aims to teach adequate heterosocial skills. (Barlow, 1973, pp. 666–667)

More interesting than Barlow's individual case, which only recently sparked a discussion about whether this and similar publications should be retracted,[3] is the testimony of an apparent consensus among clinical experts at that time that certain kinds of sexual intercourse should be supported while others should be prevented—and that doing so actually was their professional responsibility. Psychologists or psychiatrists sometimes even transgressed the law in such research by using pornography or hiring sex workers, both illegal in some jurisdictions at that time, to find out whether their methods were "successful"; that is, whether they "instigated adequate heterosexual responses". The methods described in Barlow's quote were rather harmless compared with aversive conditioning, such as using electric shocks or substances that made people feel sick, or even brain surgery and stimulation in other studies (see Davison, 2021; Hinrichsen & Katahn, 1975; Moan & Heath, 1972).

---

[3] See, for example, "Beliefs Change", published on June 14, 2022, in *Inside Higher Ed*, at: https://www.insidehighered.com/news/2022/06/14/conversion-therapy-apology-statement-raises-questions

Like Samuel Cartwright in the nineteenth century, these physicians and scientists in the twentieth century were shaped by their society and culture (just as we are by ours right now). A precondition for treating sexual preference—or the desire to be free—medically was to understand and classify it as a medical problem. The term "homosexuality" was introduced into the medical world by the German-Austrian psychiatrist Richard von Krafft-Ebing (1840–1902) in his textbook *Psychopathia Sexualis* toward the end of the nineteenth century. The *DSM-I* of 1952 listed it in the "sexual deviation" category, a subcategory of "sociopathic personality disturbances". While there is no clear definition of "sociopathy", it suggests a pathology that deviates from or even harms society. The *DSM-II* of 1968 still considered homosexuality as a mental disorder, although no longer of the "sociopathic" kind (see Drescher, 2015; Zachar & Kendler, 2012).

At different times and places, same-sex sexual intercourse has been defined as a sin or a crime. Sometimes it was simply considered normal, and there was not even a particular term for it. Greek and Roman antiquity is frequently given as an example for that. According to the written records, the situation was more complex, however. In the Roman Empire, sexual intercourse between two adult male citizens was legally prohibited. Penetrating such a person's body was simply "not done". The same goes for corporal punishment, with few exceptions in the military—and then only by an officer, the centurion, with a special vine stick. What we nowadays would call homosexual intercourse still occurred because not all men, based on their age or social status, were citizens in the described sense (Walters, 1998). This also serves as another telling example of how norms shape our thoughts and behavior.

Just as informative as the pathologization of homosexuality is its subsequent depathologization. A precondition for this was not only the growing social pressure against psychiatry by activists, but also a new definition of mental disorders requiring them to be "associated with either subjective distress or generalized impaired social effectiveness" (Friedman et al., 1976, p. 58). One of these authors, Robert L. Spitzer (1932–2015), also chaired the development of the *DSM-III* published in 1980. This was the first edition from which homosexuality was removed, after board members of the American Psychiatric Association (APA) had voted in 1973 and 1974 that it should no longer be diagnosed (see also Drescher, 2015;

Zachar & Kendler, 2012).[4] We discussed the present definition of mental disorders in the *DSM-5-TR* above, where we can see that this understanding that was introduced in the 1970s, not without resistance among psychiatrists, is still the official account.

A final example in this—already lengthy—section on social constructionism is schizophrenia, but we will elaborate further on the thoughts developed thus far at the end of this chapter. Spitzer, whom we have just referred to for his contribution to depathologizing homosexuality, developed a computer program in 1968, quite exceptional at that time, to check the consistency with which schizophrenia was diagnosed in different places (Spitzer & Endicott, 1968). His results and subsequent research indicated that the disorder was understood more broadly and thus diagnosed more frequently in the US than in the UK (Cooper et al., 1972). The opposite pattern was found for affective disorders (such as depression), which seemed to be more frequently diagnosed in the UK than the US. Another study used videos of American and English patients, which had to be assessed by clinical experts in the two countries to control for possible differences in the prevalence of disorders between places (Kendell et al., 1971). The results confirmed the existence of distinct understandings of the disorders in clinical practice. To be fair, we should remember that this was before the *DSM-III* was developed, when a growing number of psychiatrists themselves had become dissatisfied with their classification system.

Nevertheless, the example illustrates, at least to a certain extent, that clinical diagnoses are in the eye of the beholder. Although the situation has improved since then, the inter-rater reliability for the present *DSM-5* diagnoses is still not perfect (Freedman et al., 2013). Experts still can and do disagree on the correct category in individual cases. For a severe diagnosis like schizophrenia, generally characterized by a combination of "negative symptoms" (such as cognitive decline) and "positive symptoms" (positive in the sense of "added", such as hearing voices or paranoia), the consequences are anything but trivial. Because the diagnostic act in itself

---

[4] That is not the whole story. The *DSM-III* contained the category "ego-dystonic sexual orientation/homosexuality". While this did not label the same-sex sexual preference in itself a disorder, it still pathologized the suffering from a sexual orientation at odds with one's self-image. This was later removed in the revised *DSM-III-R* of 1987. In theory, a classification such as "sexual disorder not otherwise specified" since the *DSM-IV* of 1994 provides a category for diagnosing a wide range of sex-related problems when the clinical professional deems it useful.

can have a devastating impact on patients, some clinicians would like to replace the category with something less stigmatizing and to instead indicate a spectrum of psychosis risk, which all people have to some extent (see, for example, Tebartz van Elst, 2021; Van Os, 2016; Van Os & Linscott, 2012).

Uncertainty about the diagnostic entity, from Kraepelin's *dementia praecox*, later replaced with "schizophrenia" by the Swiss psychiatrist Paul E. Bleuler (1857–1939), and perhaps soon to be replaced by something else, partially explains how the category could be abused by (mostly white male) psychiatrists in the US in order to counteract riots by (mostly black male) activists of the civil rights movement of the 1950s and 1960s. Based on archive studies, Jonathan M. Metzl, Professor of Sociology and Psychiatry at Vanderbilt University in Nashville, Tennessee, described "How Schizophrenia Became a Black Disease" in that period (Metzl, 2010). As late as 1974, an advertisement in the *Archives of General Psychiatry* (now: *JAMA Psychiatry*), the official psychiatric journal of the American Medical Association, entitled "Assaultive and belligerent?" showed an angry-looking black man and proposed Haldol, a fast-acting tranquillizer, as a psychopharmacological solution: "Cooperation often begins with HALDOL", the ad explains. Could *Frauengold*, which we discussed in the preface, have been inspired by such advertisements? In any case, the same tranquilizer was still mentioned almost 50 years later in a critical reflection on structural racism in psychiatry when dealing with homeless people, the Black Lives Matter movement, and the COVID-19 pandemic (Dykema, 2021).

This section is by no means intended to detract from the contribution of clinical psychologists, psychiatrists, or other healthcare personnel, who are often the last resort for people with severe mental problems, nor to suggest that they are all racists. But it should be clear by now that essentialism or something very similar does not work as a theoretical framework for mental health and that there are at least some strong cases for social constructionism. Importantly, this does not render the mental disorder concept entirely arbitrary, as fictively illustrated in Machado de Assis's *The Alienist*.

This chapter has so far emphasized that mental health is strongly associated with cultural and social norms. We can thus take the established psychiatric disorder categories—representing the consensus of influential American psychiatrists and not "hard" or "objective" natural categories— somewhat less seriously in the remainder of the book. This will eventually also enable a broader view on substance use. But before addressing this, we shall first round off the philosophical account on "How to make sense of things" with the third and last view, pragmatism, as well as learn some basic facts about addiction and reflect on some recent diagnostic trends in the following sections.

Pragmatism

Pragmatism is the ideal stance for those who do not like complicated philosophical discussions. Put simply, it holds that we should just do "what works". In science at large, it suggests that researchers' theories and entities are the tools they use to do their work rather than necessarily reflecting something in an observer-independent "world out there", as demanded by realism (see also Chalmers, 2013). Because pragmatism comes with minimal philosophical commitments, it does not really oppose the previous views but rather shifts the perspective on the utility of a classification system or of research and clinical practice.

This in itself does not give us a clear answer as to *whom* the mental healthcare system should work for. That answer is not as obvious as one might think. Peter Zachar has advocated a pragmatic view to "help us meet scientific and professional goals, such as reliable diagnosis, prognostication, treatment selection or identification of genetic risk" (Kendler et al., 2011, p. 1146). This stance implies patients' interests, as they seek help to find solutions for their psychological problems. But health insurance providers are also stakeholders in that system and might—and in many cases actually do—limit diagnostic procedures and treatment selection to control costs.

Clinicians and scientists, in turn, are often embedded in certain institutions with their own rules and interests, such as fulfilling career and budget aims. Corrado Barbui, a much-cited depression researcher collaborating with the WHO, noted that the category major depressive disorder (MDD) "fulfils more a formal requirement than a clinical need, in particular that of being accountable and that of being coherent" (Barbui, 2015, p. 465). Simply due to their present dominance, views akin to essentialism are very useful for scientists wishing to secure research funds and publish their findings in highly competitive contexts. But, according to critical voices even from within psychiatry, that comes at the cost of neglecting therapeutic innovation and thus also patients' interests (Lewis-Fernandez et al., 2016).

This variety of possibilities illustrates that even from a pragmatic point of view some value judgments are necessary to decide whose interests should be guiding or how to define and measure utility. Obviously, the entire healthcare system would not make sense without the *patients*, the individuals that it is meant to help or heal. This can be taken as an argument for their interests being prioritized. But the innovative research on the new concept of health discussed in the introduction has also shown that different stakeholders—such as patients, clinicians, administrators, and politicians—differ in their views on what belongs to health and what does not (Huber et al., 2016). The necessity to choose and define emphasizes the fact that pragmatism, even if it comes with fewer commitments, is not an entirely neutral position either.

Providing an informed answer to all these questions goes beyond the scope of this book. But with what we have learned so far, we can now understand the *DSM* in a more meaningful way. The fact that it has avoided strong commitments about the causes of mental disorders since the *DSM-III*, that it emphasizes subjective suffering and functional impairment, and that it also seeks to improve consistency among clinical experts—what Barbui called "coherence" in the above quote—fits very well with pragmatism. The APA's diagnostic manual thus adopts a very pragmatic view. This makes a lot of sense for clinical experts who often have to take immediate action and cannot postpone their decisions until a distant future when the philosophical debates about essentialism and social constructionism may have been settled. This interim conclusion will also be useful for the next section on addiction.

2.2   What Is Addiction?

The common meaning or etymology of a term does not necessarily reflect its present clinical or scientific use, but clinicians and scientists also rely on their common language or derive terms from it. To a certain extent, their work is thus also a language praxis. As we discussed in detail in the previous sections, they use classification systems to structure what they are doing in order to provide and create consistency. Ultimately, they record their findings in written reports or publications. It can thus be useful to have background knowledge about a term's general use and origins.

The *Oxford Dictionary of English* (online edition) defines "addiction" as "the fact or condition of being addicted to a particular substance or activity". This of course shifts the question to the meaning of "addicted".

The dictionary defines this as being "physically and mentally dependent on a particular substance". "Dependence", in turn, means "the state of relying on or being controlled by someone or something else". We have thus gone from addiction to dependence to being externally controlled. The English term "addiction", derived from Latin *addicere* (literally: to speak to), originally referred to an attachment that could have been perceived as positive or negative, depending on its object, such as religious belief or gambling (Rosenthal & Faris, 2019). By contrast, the German *Sucht* relates to pathology (*siech sein*, being sick) and the Dutch *verslaving* literally expresses the notion of enslavement. The latter can be linked back to *addicere*, also used as a legal term in Roman law as early as the fifth century BCE to attach slaves to their masters (ibid.).

So what about the more technical use of the word? An influential source from the time of alcohol prohibition in the US (1920–1933) gives the following answer in a section entitled "What Drug Addiction Is":

> What, then, is the thing we call drug addiction? It is one of the anomalies of medicine, of research, of science, of religion, of social work that this subject has received so little analytical study that even after hundreds of years of addiction [...] no one knows exactly how these habit-forming drugs accomplish their fell purpose in the human body. One thing we do know, and that is that drug addiction is a habit, that it breaks down character and cripples the soul. (Graham-Mulhall, 1926, p. 95)

This quote comes from *Opium, the Demon Flower*, a book quite literally illustrating the demonization of drug use that we will discuss in more detail in Chap. 4. The work was praised in a review in *The Journal of Education* of September 13,1926 for "promoting so noble a cause", and the reviewer concluded that it should be made available "in every school and professional library in America". That recommendation seems to have been effective, as the book's third edition was already printed in 1928. The author, Sara Graham-Mulhall, had formerly been first deputy commissioner at the Department of Narcotic Drug Control of New York State and was president of the Narcotic Drug Control League at the time that *The Demon Flower* was published. She also won the *Pictorial Review* award, a grant of $5000 (corresponding to about $90,000 today) offered by the popular women's magazine to the American woman "who made the most valuable contribution to the advancement of human welfare" in a particular year.[5] Graham-Mulhall promised to use the funds to support the anti-narcotic movement. In her book, she characterized the psychology of the drug addict as follows:

> The addict loses power of concentration, power of application, power of will and the power of clear focus on ethical and moral values. He does not do this willfully. It is done for him by the drug, no matter what mental and moral fiber he may have had before taking the drug. The addict, deprived of his drug, exhibits the same psychology as a drowning rat or a drowning man. He grabs at a straw. He has then but one instinct, and that is self-preservation, which to him means drug. [...] There is no such thing in the category of addiction as a self-controlled addict. If you are taking drugs, it is automatically certain that you are prepared to lie or steal or use physical violence to get the drug you think you need. (ibid., pp. 98, 107)

The author conveniently split the world into good and evil. For her, drugs obviously belonged to the latter category. An unfortunate feature of Graham-Mulhall's writing is the amalgamation of factual statements with moral attitudes in a way that makes it difficult for the reader to distinguish between the two and to note the strong bias in her views. If we want to interpret this in a charitable way, we can imagine that in her official function she mostly became acquainted with severe cases of drug use, people whose consumption had been noticed by and then came under purview of the authorities. But some 100 years later, we know that even for hard drugs usually only a minority of users become addicted, and that this depends not only on the substance but also on social and personal factors. Let us discuss this important question in more detail.

How Likely Is Dependence?

Lee Nelken Robins (1922–2009), Professor of Social Science in Psychiatry at Washington University in St Louis, studied the drug use of US soldiers during the Vietnam War (1955–1975) and after their return. This was a unique historical opportunity to see what happened when a large number of people (mostly young men) entered a harsh environment where high-quality drugs were available in large quantities and then returned to "normal" society. According to Robins' data, based on self-reports, military

---

[5] According to the *Margaret Sanger Papers Project*, online at https://sangerpapers.wordpress.com/2011/07/08/the-company-she-kept-1924/

documents and urine tests, the prevalence of opiate use (opium and/or heroin) increased from 11% pre-Vietnam to 43% in the war zone (Robins et al., 1974). The essential question, also from a public health perspective, was how many veterans would later continue to use drugs in their home country. If Graham-Mulhall's perspective were accurate, that figure would have to be close to 43%. However, the post-Vietnam prevalence of drug consumption fell to 10% and was thus roughly equal to the lifetime prevalence of opiate use in the general population (Hall & Weier, 2017; Robins et al., 1974). But more importantly, only 1% of veterans became re addicted to heroin in the first year after their return.

The studies by Robins and her colleagues were met with disbelief because their data did not correspond to the common negative views about the substance and the results of domestic studies in the US. However, they and other researchers kept pointing out that opiate use was less stigmatized in Vietnam and that the drugs were easily available there, even of better quality and at a lower cost (Hall & Weier, 2017; Robins, 1993). This allowed most soldiers to smoke or sniff heroin rather than inject it. But because the purity was much lower and the price much higher in the US, domestic users had to inject it to achieve a similar effect. And this way of administering the substance is much more frequently associated with dependence than smoking or sniffing.

Furthermore, poorly educated men from urban areas and socially disadvantaged families with a history of drug use were more likely to both use heroin *and* become addicted in the US, whereas also other groups of men tried out the drug in Vietnam. After their return, most of the latter switched to cannabis and alcohol, more widely available and more socially accepted substances in their home country at that time (Hall & Weier, 2017). The fact that only a minority of users becomes addicted and that the likelihood depends on psychosocial factors—such as the character of an environment and social stress—is backed up by recent and experimental research (see Ahmed et al., 2020).

For example, the trials conducted by Bruce K. Alexander in the late 1970s that became widely known as *The Rat Park Experiments* illustrated how rodents, after being accustomed to opiates in cramped and environmentally deprived cages, would eschew the drugs even when sweetened with sugar after they had been moved to the much more diverse and stimulating "Rat Park" (see Gage & Sumnall, 2019). Though some criticized these trials as oversimplified, newer epidemiological data of humans suggest that 15% of the users of illegal substances become dependent (Anthony et al., 1994), and recent laboratory experiments showed that 20% of genetically very similar rats became addicted to cocaine (Lüscher et al., 2020).[6]

The conclusion is always the same: Drug dependence seems to be a biopsychosocial phenomenon that cannot merely be reduced to the features of a substance or the genes of a consumer alone. This emphasizes how complex an issue addiction is. It is also highly moralized and politicized. In 1971, decades after the Prohibition in the US but a few years before the US army withdrew from Vietnam, President Richard Nixon would declare the "War on Drugs". When his Republican successor President George H. W. Bush proclaimed the "Decade of the Brain" almost 20 years later, addiction would be identified as one of the top priorities for the neurosciences:

> Research may also prove valuable in our war on drugs, as studies provide greater insight into how people become addicted to drugs and how drugs affect the brain. These studies may also help produce effective treatments for chemical dependency and help us to understand and prevent the harm done to the preborn children of pregnant women who abuse drugs and alcohol.[7]

The DSM on Addiction

This was in 1990. But how does the present DSM characterize addiction? The DSM-5-TR contains a section on "Substance-Related and Addictive Disorders" (APA, 2022). It distinguishes "use disorders", acute intoxication, and withdrawal for several substances (e.g. alcohol, caffeine, or cannabis) or substance classes (e.g. hallucinogens, opioids, or stimulants). The "use disorders" generally contain a list of symptoms referring to loss of control (e.g. consuming more than wanted or in spite of negative individual or social effects) or psychological processes such as tolerance and

---

[6] Measuring this precisely presumes a clear understanding of what addiction is, but this section shows that there is not an unambiguous answer. However, the online Addiction Center based in Orlando Florida, which can hardly be accused of downplaying drug harms, states that "about 10%" of people misusing prescription opioids and "roughly 10%" of all cannabis users become addicted; no such figures are provided for alcohol, cocaine, hallucinogens, heroin, methamphetamine, and nicotine; see: https://www.addictioncenter.com/addiction/addiction-statistics/

[7] Presidential Proclamation 6158 of July 17, 1990, online at https://www.loc.gov/loc/brain/proclaim.html

craving. The section's introduction explains that "the phrase 'drug addiction' is not applied as a diagnostic term in this classification, although it is in common usage in many countries to describe severe problems related to compulsive and habitual use of substances."

Besides these substance-related categories, the section contains one notable deviation: *gambling disorder*. This single exception probably explains the "...and Addictive Disorders" of the title. According to the manual, this reflects "evidence that gambling behaviors activate reward systems similar to those activated by drugs of abuse and that produce some behavioral symptoms that appear comparable to those produced by the substance use disorders". We shall get back to the point about the reward systems shortly. Apart from what we have discussed so far, the roughly 80,000 words of the *DSM*'s section on substance use and addictive disorders (for comparison: the whole present book has fewer than 50,000 words) contain the term "addiction" only *five* times in the body of the text. And these very few places often create the impression that the editors forgot to replace the term with the more common expression "substance use disorder". In conclusion, the *DSM* seems to eschew "addiction" as much as possible, perhaps because there is no generally accepted definition.

Two Pragmatic Views

As we have learned above, such situations call for pragmatic solutions. I summarize two approaches to assessing alcohol dependence in Box 2.1, the one developed by the German Cancer Research Center (Schaller et al., 2017) and the Alcohol Use Disorders Identification Test (AUDIT) of the World Health Organization (WHO).[8] These approaches provide us with a clearer notion of what dependence is and why it can become a problem. Many of these aspects can be generalized to other substances as well.

We may thus conclude pragmatically that addiction or dependence is a complex condition combining (1) someone's psycho-behavioral loss of control, (2) impaired daily functioning such as the failure to pursue other interests, (3) psychological processes like craving, desire, or compulsion, and (4) psycho-physiological processes such as developing tolerance or withdrawal effects. It should be stressed that dependence often arises through a psychological learning or coping mechanism: People may use a

[8] Online at https://www.who.int/publications/i/item/WHO-MSD-MSB-01.6a

Box 2.1   Assessing Dependence

The German Cancer Research Center uses the following six criteria to assess alcohol dependence:

1. Do you have a strong desire or compulsion to consume the substance?
2. Tolerance: Do you need larger quantities of the substance to achieve an effect?
3. Do you continue to consume in spite of health damage due to the substance use?
4. Do you have difficulty controlling the beginning, the end, or the quantity of the consumption?
5. Do you have withdrawal effects when consuming less or nothing of the substance? (Such as trembling, unrest, sweating, sleeping problems, circulatory problems, cramps, or confusion.)
6. Do you increasingly neglect other interests due to the substance use?

According to these researchers, an alcohol dependence syndrome is present when at least three of the six criteria have persisted simultaneously during the previous 12 months. Note that I have deliberately replaced "alcohol" with the more general "substance use", as this model can be meaningfully applied to other drugs as well. The WHO's AUDIT uses ten items instead to calculate a score from 0 to 40 points. The higher the score, the more likely that an alcohol use disorder is present. To assess someone's precise score, the original version should be used. I summarize the items here to illustrate the idea behind drug dependence or addiction, again replacing "alcohol" with "substance". As with the previous list, the questions usually refer to the previous 12 months:

1. How often and what quantities of the substance do you typically consume?
2. How often were you unable to stop using the substance once you had started?

(continued)

Box 2.1   (continued)

3. How often have you failed to do what was expected of you because of the substance use?
4. How often did you need to take the substance in the morning to get yourself going after a session of heavy use?
5. How often did you have a feeling of guilt or remorse after using the substance?
6. How often have you been unable to remember what happened the night before because of substance use?
7. Have you or has someone else been injured as a result of your substance use?
8. Has someone been concerned about your substance use or suggested that you cut down?

One notable difference is the WHO's stronger reliance on subjective factors. For example, if people do not experience blackouts, feel no remorse, and can hide their use successfully from others, then that already eliminates 12 of the 40 points, or 30% of the maximum score. People with responses suggesting a dependency according to any of the lists should consider talking to a medical, a psychological, or a social professional about their substance use.

substance to suppress unwanted thoughts or feelings (e.g., the research on soldiers in Vietnam summarized above named dealing with boredom, homesickness, and disturbed sleep) or to achieve a desired experience (e.g., feeling high, euphoric, or connected with others).

Increasing positive or decreasing negative feelings both act as a reward, a reinforcer raising the likelihood of substance use in the future. This is particularly likely when a drug directly activates the brain's reward systems, as the *DSM* explained with respect to gambling disorder. After a sufficient number of repetitions, users may have learned that they need the particular substance (or activity) to achieve the desired state and in this sense have become dependent. In the next section, comparing gambling with some other conditions will allow us to understand some recent diagnostic trends in the domain of mental health.

2.3   RECENT DIAGNOSTIC TRENDS

We have seen above that the APA added gambling disorder to the DSM as the only nonsubstance-related addictive disorder, sometimes also called a "behavioral addiction", on the grounds that it activates the brain's reward systems. This seems to lend the category some neurobiological credibility. Two interesting psychosocial symptoms of that disorder's nine criteria are, firstly, gambling when feeling distressed and, secondly, relying on the help of others, particularly their money, "to relieve desperate financial situations caused by gambling" (APA, 2022).

It is known for decades that there are social causes for the former, distress, such as poverty or being a single parent (Mirowsky & Ross, 2012). The latter, relying on help, is remarkable in that very rich people thus have lower odds of being diagnosed with gambling disorder, simply because they have enough money. We can again understand these aspects from a pragmatic perspective in combination with social constructionism: People whose loss of control over their gambling gets them into financial trouble will be more likely to seek help; and the *DSM*'s criteria reflect the consensus of psychiatrists who then see such people more frequently in their clinical work.

A "behavioral addiction" that has not made it into the DSM so far is *internet gaming disorder*. It was only added to the appendix under "Conditions for Further Study" because "research on these and other behavioral syndromes is less clear" (APA, 2022). The authors specify that "[t]his disorder is distinct from Internet gambling, which is included under gambling disorder". This distinction will be challenging for psychiatrists in the future, since so-called loot boxes in computer games, with which the gaming industry earns billions, strongly resemble gambling and are therefore starting to be regulated as such in some countries.[9] These in-game mechanisms offer random special features against payment, as in a lottery.

Yet, the WHO experts drew a different conclusion and have already added *gaming disorder* to the new ICD-11. The International Classification of Diseases (ICD) is the WHO's statistical and diagnostic manual, and countries not using the DSM commonly employ the ICD's section for

---

[9] Since 2018, Belgium and the Netherlands have considered games involving loot boxes as gambling, such that the providers would require a special license. Apparently, these rules are enforced with mixed success, see: https://arstechnica.com/gaming/2022/05/loot-box-laws-block-diablo-immortal-launch-in-some-european-countries/

mental disorders instead. As with gambling, the findings that gaming activates the brain's reward systems played a significant role in the WHO's decision. The category has already been intensively investigated by scientists, some of whom are even looking for medical treatments (see, for example, Bae et al., 2018; Starcevic & Khazaal, 2020; Stavropoulos et al., 2019).

We thus see once more that leading psychiatrists can and indeed do disagree about what should be considered a valid diagnostic category. In countries relying on the ICD for the domain of mental health, gaming disorder is now becoming an official medical classification. This has real implications for people's lives, in this case particularly young men, who are the most active gamers. In line with what we have discussed earlier in this chapter, a loss of control reflected in diminished interest in other activities and facing social difficulties is a central aspect of the new disorder. But we should hesitate to medicalize our moral beliefs. For example, Joost A. M. Meerloo (1903–1976), a Dutch physician and psychoanalyst who flew to England during the Second World War and emigrated to the US in 1950, wrote about *television addiction* (Meerloo, 1954). He was particularly concerned about the use of this new medium among children and teenagers and concluded "[t]hat television fascination is a real addiction, that is to say, television can become a habit-forming device, the influence of which cannot be stopped without active therapeutic interference" (ibid., p. 291).

Such examples draw our attention to other possible "behavioral addictions", such as exercise, Instagram, or sex addiction. Some clinicians and researchers are arguing in favor of the introduction of these and many more similar categories. Even the existence of an "Argentinian tango addiction" has been investigated (see Rosenthal & Faris, 2019). We can imagine that people must experience activities that they engage in for many hours without external pressure as rewarding, and that some individuals are excessively active such that negative consequences ensue. Using a broad definition of "addiction", including controversial categories such as "food addiction" or "work addiction", Sussman and colleagues concluded that 47% of adults might be addicted to something within a 12-month period (Sussman et al., 2011). We see once more how much depends on how disorders are defined and how researchers subsequently measure them.

Is the Prevalence of Mental Disorders Increasing?

This raises the broader question of whether mental disorders are generally becoming more prevalent. It should be clear by now that the answer is not trivial as—unlike beans in a jar—there is no observer-independent way of counting these entities. The high number of news reports on mental health initially suggests an affirmative answer. A less arbitrary measure is the relative frequency with which the topic is covered in books (Fig. 2.1). However, this could simply mean that it is attracting more attention while the prevalence of the actual disorders remains more or less the same.

So what answer do researchers give, in particular epidemiologists who are specialized in investigating the prevalence of disorders and diseases in the population? Allow me first a historical remark: Our present question was already hotly debated in the 1960s. Figure 2.1 indeed shows a growing interest in mental health at that time. One particularly controversial

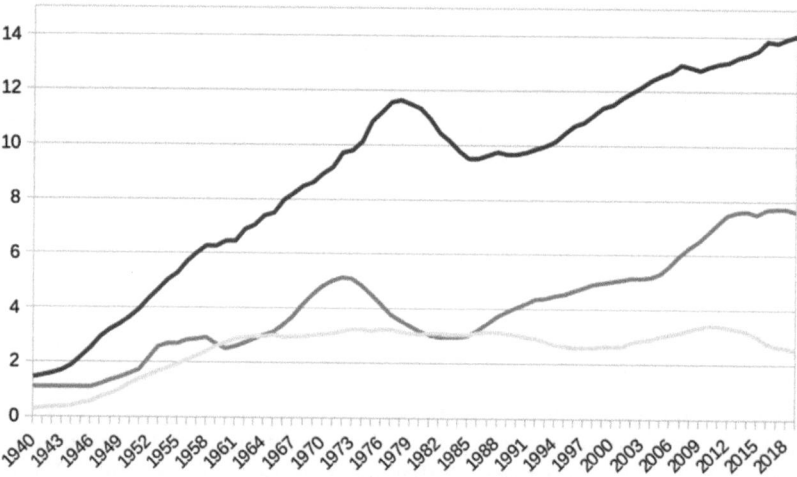

Fig. 2.1 More Attention Paid to Mental Health. Mental health has increasingly been addressed in books published in English since the Second World War (*blue line*), with a first peak in the late 1970s. Writing about addiction has also become more common (*red line*), with a first peak in the early 1970s. By contrast, steroids (*yellow line*), which are used to change one's body (see Chap. 4), have not become more common a topic in English-language books since the 1960s (*yellow line*). Source: Google Ngram (lines smoothed; ×10⁶)

issue was whether people living in urban environments had more psychological problems than those from rural places. Thus, when the results of 1911 representative interviews for the Midtown Manhattan Study were published in 1962, suggesting that 81.5% of citizens had mental health issues, many understood this as supporting the hypothesis that cities are an unhealthy environment for humans (Srole et al., 1962).

However, we can see upon closer inspection that this very high percentage included people with very mild issues who probably did not need the support of an expert. Remember the "clinical significance", "subjective suffering", and "functional impairment" conditions discussed above. It is important to know that the symptom severity of the interviewees in Manhattan was rated on a scale from 0 to 6. If we take a more realistic cut-off value (e.g., a severity of 3 and higher), then 23.4% of the citizens would count as having a mental disorder, based on the same data. This would also be more consistent with the recent surveys we will discuss shortly and shows that such values cannot be interpreted meaningfully without background information on how they are calculated.

A much-cited analysis of the mental health of the inhabitants of 30 European countries reported figures halfway between the percentages that we have just discussed (Wittchen et al., 2011). Again based on representative interviews, these researchers estimated a 12-month prevalence of at least one mental disorder of 38.2%. This means that more than a third of the population would meet the criteria within any given year! It is important to know that this was based on a selection of only 27 common disorders, while the DSM distinguishes several hundred. But carrying out representative interviews about so many categories simply is not manageable using this epidemiological approach. Thus, we can only speculate that the overall prevalence would probably be above 40%, perhaps even higher than 50%, if all DSM disorders were included.

We have also just discussed a study that estimated the 12-month prevalence of addiction in the US adult population at 47%, using an exceptionally broad understanding of the category (Sussman et al., 2011). Combining their approach with that of the epidemiologists summarized in the previous paragraph would yield an incredibly high prevalence of mental disorders. Remembering the lesson we learned from The Alienist at the beginning of the chapter, we may then well ask whether deviance from the norm is in fact the new norm if it is so common.

It is particularly noteworthy that when the principal investigators of the huge epidemiological study repeated their survey for Germany alone, they reported a much lower 12-month prevalence of 27.7% (Jacobi et al., 2014). The researchers explained this difference by the fact that fewer disorders were included. But if the results are so very dependent on the scientists' methodological choices, they are not very informative about the "real" prevalence. Another caveat is that the interviewees in such studies are commonly asked to report from memory any symptoms within the past year. This not only has limited reliability but is also not very indicative of the clinical significance of the psychological problems as explained above.

If we understand such figures to literally represent people in need of psychological or psychiatric services, the mental health system would simply collapse. Accordingly, the study found that of the interviewees who fulfilled the criteria for one mental disorder, only 11% reported having sought help (Jacobi et al., 2014). Besides the unfortunate fact that some people with very severe problems do not seek or receive the help they need, this finding strongly suggests that most of the people identified in such epidemiological studies do not perceive themselves as being truly impaired and prefer to solve their problems on their own.

A similar epidemiological study investigating the issue globally reported a 12-month prevalence of at least one mental disorder of 17.6% and a lifetime prevalence of 29.2% (Steel et al., 2014). While these findings still suggest that almost one in five people require psychological or psychiatric help at least once every year, epidemiologists are often quick to deny that there is any increase. That people suffer more from psychological problems is frequently assumed in the context of a social-political critique. But how can epidemiologists deny this with certainty if their methods and results differ so much? Besides, reviews and analyses focusing on individual disorders, such as ADHD (Thomas et al., 2015) or anxiety disorders (Remes et al., 2016), *do* report increasing prevalences as well as variability between countries and different editions of diagnostic manuals. To add a final complexity, there are in fact epidemiological studies reporting an increase in mental disorders on the global level, though their figures cannot fully explain the increased amount of diagnoses we see for many diagnoses (Richter et al., 2019).

In any case, there is no simple answer to the question posed in this section. Unlike counting the beans in a jar, the situation for mental disorders is rather like counting without knowing precisely what a bean is, with people occasionally adding or removing beans, with a few beans turning into peas, and with a couple of lentils becoming beans. Imagine what that would mean for the chemical elements: Gold, for example, would turn out to be mercury instead. Many instances of what researchers considered to be helium was later defined as hydrogen. Chlorine proved not to be elementary at all and was thus removed from the list while experts finally agreed on adding "hypertine" (something I've just made up).

New Disorders

We discussed in a previous section how complex it is to define addiction. But the same goes for many other disorders: There has been a long discussion about the distinction between depression and grief after bereavement (see Frances, 2013; Zachar et al., 2017). This question has now been settled by the APA with the introduction of *prolonged grief disorder* into *the DSM-5-TR*, in the event that a clinical expert deems a client's grief to be culturally inappropriate (APA, 2022). *Gender dysphoria* has replaced *gender identity disorder* since the *DSM-5*, as psychiatrists believed it to be less stigmatizing a category; it may eventually be removed from the manual altogether. Some clinicians and scientists are trying to have *orthodoxia nervosa* included, excessive discipline concerning food, or to have *sluggish cognitive tempo* (which others have since called *concentration deficit disorder*) recognized as a new subtype of ADHD. There were more historical examples in much more detail in the section on social constructionism.

The point should be sufficiently clear by now. Now that all these complex arguments and facts have been presented, it is time to conclude this chapter and make a constructive suggestion as to what mental disorders are. We will continue to discuss a related question later in the book, where we recognize that—while epidemiologists disagree on the issue—data from studies investigating actual medical practice unmistakably report a strong increase in the diagnosis of mental disorders, which then also often implies the prescription of psychopharmacological drugs.

2.4   Interim Conclusion: Mental Disorders Are Not Things

The best way to summarize all of the above would be: *Mental disorders are not things!* Ian Hacking described them as "moving targets" (Hacking, 1999). Clinicians and scientists, along with other social institutions, sometimes "make up" a certain way of being a person, and people thus classified and described often adapt in such a way that a "looping effect" occurs. Remember the analogy with the beans in a jar. Hacking convincingly described this for *multiple personality disorder* (MPD) in the 1980s:

When psychiatrists started diagnosing a few sensational cases in the 1970s, they also attracted considerable media coverage (see Harris, 2011; Nathan, 2011; Schreiber, 1973). Subsequently, more and more people manifested the symptoms. Not only did they become more bizarre, but the number of patients' "personalities" increased within a decade from 2 or 3 on average to 17 (Hacking, 1995). The disorder was also merchandized: Some patients literally sold their story, an MPD board game was produced, and "split bars" opened in some cities where people could meet such patients or where people with an MPD diagnosis could get to know each other. Over time, the diagnostic criteria changed again and again until the *DSM-IV* of 1994 eventually replaced MPD with *dissociative identity disorder*.

As I have repeatedly stressed in this chapter, this does not make mental disorders any less real. Even if a target is moving, it is still a target! But this dooms to failure any efforts to describe their "essence". The same goes for attempts to reduce them to biological states such as gene expression or brain states, on which billions are still spent every year. It just does not make sense to *reify* mental disorders, to describe them as things, if they are massively heterogeneous and dynamic processes, which are also culturally mediated. The outcome of almost 200 years of research supports this view, even for those disorders judged by clinicians to have mostly biological causes (Ahn et al., 2009; Fig. 2.2).

According to my own theoretical research, mental disorders *are* and *are not* brain disorders: They are in the sense that all our psychological processes are embodied, just as your current reading is enabled by a certain neural and body structure and the meaning of this sentence is somehow represented in your network of billions of neurons and other cells with their connections and activities; they are not because they are not things, and psychological language cannot be reduced to biological terms (Schleim, 2022a; see also Frisch, 2016; Fuchs, 2018; Moncrieff, 2020). The "neural correlates" or genes allegedly associated with the disorders reflect only some transient and limited statistical aspects of people's experiences or behaviors (Schleim & Roiser, 2009). And these findings actually often fail to be replicated: Based on data from tens of thousands of people, sometimes even more than a hundred thousand, we now know that genetic variability explains almost nothing in the domain of mental health (Giangrande et al., 2022) and also that neuroimaging is coming increasingly under fire (see Marek et al., 2022). When we do the maths and realize that, for example, the present *DSM* criteria for ADHD allow for

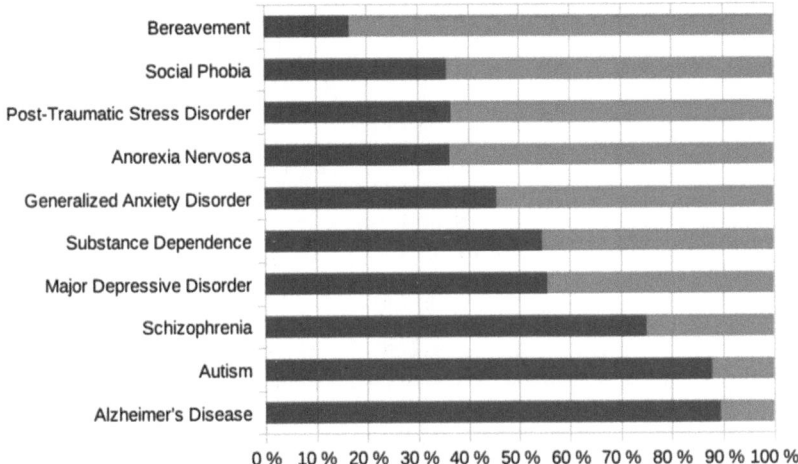

Fig. 2.2 Clinicians' Beliefs About Causes. Ahn and colleagues (2009) asked clinical experts (n = 89) to rate the causes of a subset of *DSM-IV* disorders as biological or psychological on a scale from 1 to 5. The following list shows a simplified selection of their results, illustrating how biological (*blue*) or psychological (*red*) the experts on average rated these disorders. These results strongly correlated with the view as to whether medication or psychotherapy would be the best treatment

116,220 different valid expressions of the disorder, we can better understand why the results must be as they are (Schleim, 2022a).

Many scientists are tricked by the application of statistical methods that provide only a transitory snapshot of something common to a selected group of patients while neglecting the individual heterogeneity and diversity of real life. But even without complex calculations and argumentation, it should be clear that, firstly, the very abstract and consensus-based disorder categories sanctioned by influential experts who, secondly, use a formalized technical language of symptoms are not the same as people's actual experiences, behaviors, and physiological processes (Fig. 2.3). Added to that is the historical and cultural variability (see Watters, 2010), which also shows that people learn to express their sensations, thoughts, problems, and situations in a certain kind of language. In our present time and situation, this has often become the language of clinical psychology and psychiatry, culturally disseminated by the media. In some non-Western cultures, though, it is much more common to describe one's distress in

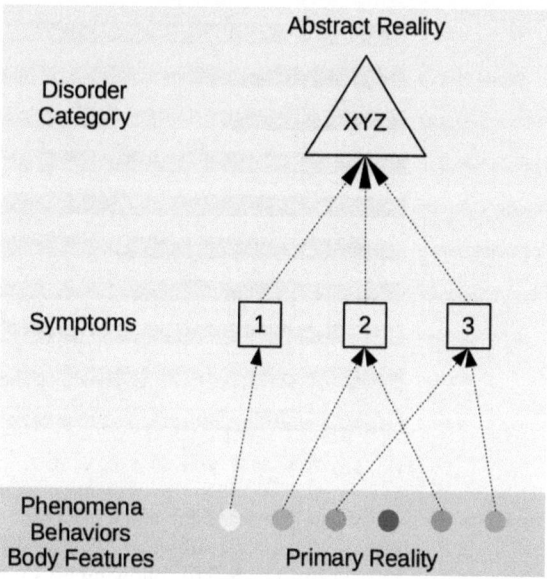

Fig. 2.3 Psychological Problems and Language. Someone's experiences ("phenomena"), behaviors, and body features are part of what I call here "primary reality". Although experiences can be psychosocially complex and culturally mediated, they exist more independently of an expert's description. For example, in the case of a depressive episode, this could involve someone not falling asleep easily, engaging in excessive physical exercise, losing weight without dieting, and experiencing a bad mood or feelings of guilt. When clinicians and scientists speak of "symptoms", they begin formalizing such processes and states of the primary reality in their technical language. An abstract, consensus-based disorder category such as major depressive disorder (MDD) eventually collects particular symptoms in a pragmatic way. The *DSM-5* criteria for MDD then allow 227 unique symptom combinations, which can, however, be based on an indefinite variability in primary reality

bodily terms (Antić, 2021; Desai & Chaturvedi, 2017; Nichter, 2010), and some psychiatrists are trying intensively to get body and environment back "inside" psychotherapy (see Fuchs, 2018; Van der Kolk, 2014).

This standpoint by no means denies the reality or severity of conditions like those that clinicians nowadays call "schizophrenia", nor that psychopharmacology or other brain-based treatments can be helpful in dealing with the symptoms. There is no contradiction here because my own and similar accounts do not deny the embodiment of our perception, cognition, emotion, and behavior (see also Schleim, 2020, 2022b). It further deserves mentioning here that people who hear voices, for example, can find nonmedical ways of dealing with their experiences (see McCarthy-Jones, 2012) and that patients with some severe diagnoses have better prognoses in countries that are less committed to biomedical treatments (Margraf & Schneider, 2016). A recent review furthermore found a total of 34 different models in the scientific literature that sought to make sense of people's psychological problems (Richter & Dixon, 2022). There are thus many good reasons to believe that the prevailing account is not the last word.

Much more can be said about mental disorders and the mental health system, as has in fact been done elsewhere (e.g., Frances, 2013; Scull, 2022). Nikolas Rose, for example, concluded in his comprehensive book on *Our Psychiatric Future* that while ever more people are experiencing psychological distress, many of them should be helped by community-based services rather than psychiatric labeling and medical treatment (Rose, 2019). Moreover, the proximal causes of this distress—such as violence, exclusion, and isolation—should be removed. This is probably all the more true during and after the coronavirus pandemic than previously.

We have now finished what is theoretically the most demanding chapter of the book. One of its primary aims has been to refute essentialism in order to enable a different view of mental health and enhancement, particularly "addiction" and substance use, which are further discussed in the following chapters. But we have actually learned much more about philosophical stances to make sense of things, about the distinction between "normal" and "abnormal" psychological processes, and about how the mental healthcare and science systems work. Essentialism would be the clearest guide for classification and treatment but it is unrealistic for mental disorders, even though they are embodied. Social constructionism emphasizes the cultural and institutional backgrounds to understand them and reminds us not to forget their psychosocial causes. And, last but not least, pragmatism emphasizes that classification systems should be useful in practical terms and that patients cannot wait until all scientific disagreement has been settled. It is helpful to keep these conclusions in mind for the remainder of the book.

References

Ahmed, S. H., Badiani, A., Miczek, K. A., & Müller, C. P. (2020). Non-pharmacological factors that determine drug use and addiction. *Neuroscience & Biobehavioral Reviews, 110*, 3–27.

Ahn, W., Proctor, C. C., & Flanagan, E. H. (2009). Mental health clinicians' beliefs about the biological, psychological, and environmental bases of mental disorders. *Cognitive Science, 33*, 147–182.

Anderson, M. L., Kinnison, J., & Pessoa, L. (2013). Describing functional diversity of brain regions and brain networks. *NeuroImage, 73*, 50–58.

Anthony, J. C., Warner, L. A., & Kessler, R. C. (1994). Comparative epidemiology of dependence on tobacco, alcohol, controlled substances, and inhalants: Basic findings from the National Comorbidity Survey. *Experimental and Clinical Psychopharmacology, 2*, 244–268.

Antić, A. (2021). Transcultural psychiatry: Cultural difference, universalism and social psychiatry in the age of decolonisation. *Culture, Medicine, and Psychiatry, 45*(3), 359–384.

APA [American Psychiatric Association]. (2022). *Diagnostic and statistical manual of mental disorders* (5th ed., text rev.). APA Press.

Bae, S., Hong, J. S., Kim, S. M., & Han, D. H. (2018). Bupropion shows different effects on brain functional connectivity in patients with internet-based gambling disorder and internet gaming disorder. *Frontiers in Psychiatry, 9*, 130.

Barbui, C. (2015). Clinical use of the diagnostic criteria for major depressive disorder. *Epidemiology and Psychiatric Sciences, 24*, 464–465.

Barlow, D. H. (1973). Increasing heterosexual responsiveness in the treatment of sexual deviation: A review of the clinical and experimental evidence. *Behavior Therapy, 4*, 655–671.

Berger, P. L., & Luckmann, T. (1966). *The social construction of reality: A treatise in the sociology of knowledge*. Anchor Books.

Bynum, W. F. (1994). *Science and the practice of medicine in the nineteenth century*. Cambridge University Press.

Cartwright, S. A. (1851). Report on the disease and physical peculiarities of the negro race. *New Orleans Medical and Surgical Journal, 7*, 691–715.

Chalmers, A. F. (2013). *What is this thing called science?* (4th ed.). Hackett Publishing Company.

Cooper, J. E., Kendell, R. E., Gurland, B. J., Sharpe, L., Copeland, J. R. M., & Simon, R. (1972). *Psychiatric diagnosis in New York and London: A comparative study of mental hospital admissions*. Oxford University Press.

Davison, K. (2021). Cold war Pavlov: Homosexual aversion therapy in the 1960s. *History of the Human Sciences, 34*, 89–119.

Desai, G., & Chaturvedi, S. K. (2017). Idioms of distress. *Journal of Neurosciences in Rural Practice, 8*, S094–S097.

Drescher, J. (2015). Out of DSM: Depathologizing homosexuality. *Behavioral Sciences, 5*, 565–575.

Dykema, L.-R. (2021). The radicalization of a white psychiatrist. *Psychiatric Services, 72*, 470–472.

Faye, J. (2019). Copenhagen Interpretation of Quantum Mechanics. In E. N. Zalta (Ed.), *The Stanford Encyclopedia of Philosophy* (Winter 2019 Edition). https://plato.stanford.edu/archives/win2019/entries/qm-copenhagen/

Follett, R. J. (2005). *The sugar masters: Planters and slaves in Louisiana's cane world, 1820–1860*. Louisiana State University Press.

Frances, A. (2013). *Saving normal: An insider's revolt against out-of-control psychiatric diagnosis, DSM-5, big pharma, and the medicalization of ordinary life*. William Morrow.

Freedman, R., Lewis, D. A., Michels, R., Pine, D. S., Schultz, S. K., Tamminga, C. A., ... & Yager, J. (2013). The initial field trials of DSM-5: New blooms and old thorns. *American Journal of Psychiatry, 170*, 1–5.

Friedman, R. C., Green, R., & Spitzer, R. L. (1976). Reassessment of homosexuality and transsexualism. *Annual Review of Medicine, 27*, 57–62.

Frisch, S. (2016). Are mental disorders brain diseases, and what does this mean? A clinical-neuropsychological perspective. *Psychopathology, 49*, 135–142.

Fuchs, T. (2018). *Ecology of the brain: The phenomenology and biology of the embodied mind*. Oxford University Press.

Gage, S. H., & Sumnall, H. R. (2019). Rat Park: How a rat paradise changed the narrative of addiction. *Addiction, 114*, 917–922.

Giangrande, E. J., Weber, R. S., & Turkheimer, E. (2022). What do we know about the genetic architecture of psychopathology? *Annual Review of Clinical Psychology, 18*, 19–42.

Gordon, J. A. (2016). On being a circuit psychiatrist. *Nature Neuroscience, 19*, 1385–1386.

Graham-Mulhall, S. (1926). *Opium, the demon flower*. Montrose Publishing Co.

Gribbin, J. (1995). *Schrödinger's kittens and the search for reality: Solving the quantum mysteries*. Little, Brown & Co.

Griesinger, W. (1845/1867). *Mental Pathology and Therapeutics* (2nd ed., Engl. transl.). The New Sydenham Society.

Hacking, I. (1995). *Rewriting the soul: Multiple personality and the sciences of memory*. Princeton University Press.

Hacking, I. (1999). *The social construction of what?* Harvard University Press.

Hall, W., & Weier, M. (2017). Lee Robins' studies of heroin use among US Vietnam veterans. *Addiction, 112*, 176–180.

Harris, B. (2011). Sybil, Inc. *Science, 334*, 312.

Hengartner, M. P. (2022). *Evidence-biased antidepressant prescription: Overmedicalisation, flawed research, and conflicts of interest*. Palgrave Macmillan.

Hinrichsen, J. J., & Katahn, M. (1975). Recent trends and new developments in the treatment of homosexuality. *Psychotherapy: Theory. Research and Practice, 12,* 83–92.

Huber, M., van Vliet, M., Giezenberg, M., Winkens, B., Heerkens, Y., Dagnelie, P., & Knottnerus, J. (2016). Towards a 'patient-centred' operationalisation of the new dynamic concept of health: A mixed methods study. *BMJ Open, 6,* e010091.

Hyman, S. E. (2007). Can neuroscience be integrated into the DSM-V? *Nature Reviews Neuroscience, 8,* 725–U716.

Hyman, S. E. (2021). Psychiatric disorders: Grounded in human biology but not natural kinds. *Perspectives in Biology and Medicine, 64,* 6–28.

Insel, T. (2010). Faulty circuits. *Scientific American, 302,* 44–51.

Jacobi, F., Höfler, M., Strehle, J., Mack, S., Gerschler, A., Scholl, L., Busch, M. A., Maske, U., Hapke, U., Gaebel, W., & Wittchen, H. U. (2014). Psychische störungen in der allgemeinbevölkerung. *Der Nervenarzt, 85,* 77–87.

Kendell, R. E., Cooper, J. E., Gourlay, A. J., Copeland, J. R. M., Sharpe, L., & Gurland, B. J. (1971). Diagnostic criteria of American and British psychiatrists. *Archives of General Psychiatry, 25,* 123–130.

Kendler, K. S. (2009). An historical framework for psychiatric nosology. *Psychological Medicine, 39,* 1935–1941.

Kendler, K. S. (2016). The nature of psychiatric disorders. *World Psychiatry, 15,* 5–12.

Kendler, K. S., Zachar, P., & Craver, C. (2011). What kinds of things are psychiatric disorders? *Psychological Medicine, 41,* 1143–1150.

Kupfer, D. J., First, M. B., & Regier, D. A. (2002). *A research agenda for DSM-V.* American Psychiatric Association.

Lewis-Fernandez, R., Rotheram-Borus, M. J., Betts, V. T., Greenman, L., Essock, S. M., Escobar, J. I., Barch, D., Hogan, M. F., Arean, P. A., Druss, B. G., & Iversen, P. (2016). Rethinking funding priorities in mental health research. *British Journal of Psychiatry, 208,* 507–509.

Lüscher, C., Robbins, T. W., & Everitt, B. J. (2020). The transition to compulsion in addiction. *Nature Reviews Neuroscience, 21,* 247–263.

Machado de Assis, J. M. (1882/2013). *The alienist and other stories of nineteenth-century Brazil* (Trans. J. C. Chasteen). Hackett Publishing Company.

Marek, S., Tervo-Clemmens, B., Calabro, F. J., Montez, D. F., Kay, B. P., Hatoum, A. S., Donohue, M. R., Foran, W., Miller, R. L., Hendrickson, T. J., & Dosenbach, N. U. F. (2022). Reproducible brain-wide association studies require thousands of individuals. *Nature, 603,* 654–660.

Margraf, J., & Schneider, S. (2016). From neuroleptics to neuroscience and from Pavlov to psychotherapy: More than just the "emperor's new treatments" for mental illnesses? *EMBO Molecular Medicine, 8,* 1115–1117.

McCarthy-Jones, S. (2012). *Hearing voices: The histories, causes, and meanings of auditory verbal hallucinations.* Cambridge University Press.

Meerloo, J. A. (1954). Television addiction and reactive apathy. *The Journal of Nervous and Mental Disease, 120,* 290–291.

Metzl, J. (2010). *The protest psychosis: How schizophrenia became a black disease.* Beacon Press.

Mirowsky, J., & Ross, C. E. (2012). *Social causes of psychological distress* (2nd ed.). AldineTransaction.

Moan, C. E., & Heath, R. G. (1972). Septal stimulation for the initiation of heterosexual behavior in a homosexual male. *Journal of Behavior Therapy and Experimental Psychiatry, 3,* 23–30.

Moncrieff, J. (2020). "It was the brain tumor that done it!": Szasz and Wittgenstein on the importance of distinguishing disease from behavior and implications for the nature of mental disorder. *Philosophy, Psychiatry, & Psychology, 27,* 169–181.

Moncrieff, J., Cooper, R. E., Stockmann, T., Amendola, S., Hengartner, M. P., & Horowitz, M. A. (2022). The serotonin theory of depression: A systematic umbrella review of the evidence. *Molecular Psychiatry,* 1–14.

Nathan, D. (2011). *Sybil exposed: The extraordinary story behind the famous multiple personality case.* Free Press.

Nichter, M. (2010). Idioms of distress revisited. *Culture, Medicine, and Psychiatry, 34,* 401–416.

Remes, O., Brayne, C., van der Linde, R., & Lafortune, L. (2016). A systematic review of reviews on the prevalence of anxiety disorders in adult populations. *Brain and Behavior, 6,* 497.

Richter, D., & Dixon, J. (2022). Models of mental health problems: A quasi-systematic review of theoretical approaches. *Journal of Mental Health,* 1–11.

Richter, D., Wall, A., Bruen, A., & Whittington, R. (2019). Is the global prevalence rate of adult mental illness increasing? Systematic review and meta-analysis. *Acta Psychiatrica Scandinavica, 140,* 393–407.

Robins, L. N. (1993). Vietnam veterans' rapid recovery from heroin addiction: A fluke or normal expectation? *Addiction, 88,* 1041–1054.

Robins, L. N., Davis, D. H., & Goodwin, D. W. (1974). Drug use by US army enlisted men in Vietnam: A follow-up on their return home. *American Journal of Epidemiology, 99,* 235–249.

Rose, N. S. (2019). *Our psychiatric future: The politics of mental health.* Polity.

Rosenthal, R. J., & Faris, S. B. (2019). The etymology and early history of 'addiction'. *Addiction Research & Theory, 27,* 437–449.

Schaller, K., Kahnert, S., & Mons, U. (2017). *Alkoholatlas Deutschland 2017.* Deutsches Krebsforschungszentrum.

Schleim, S. (2009). The risk that neurogenetic approaches may inflate the psychiatric concept of disease and how to cope with it. *Poiesis & Praxis, 6,* 79–91.

Schleim, S. (2020). To overcome psychiatric patients' mind–brain dualism, reifying the mind Won't help. *Frontiers in Psychiatry, 11,* 605.

Schleim, S. (2021). Neurorights in History: A Contemporary Review of José M. R. Delgado's "Physical Control of the Mind" (1969) and Elliot S. Valenstein's "Brain Control" (1973). *Frontiers in Human Neuroscience,* 15.

Schleim, S. (2022a). Why mental disorders are brain disorders. And why they are not: ADHD and the challenges of heterogeneity and reification. *Frontiers. Psychiatry, 13,* 943049.

Schleim, S. (2022b). Grounded in biology: Why the context-dependency of psychedelic drug effects means opportunities, not problems for anthropology and pharmacology. *Frontiers in Psychiatry, 13,* 906487.

Schleim, S., & Roiser, J. P. (2009). fMRI in translation: The challenges facing real-world applications. *Frontiers in Human Neuroscience, 3,* 63.

Schreiber, F. R. (1973). *Sybil.* Regnery.

Scull, A. (2022). *Desperate remedies: Psychiatry's turbulent quest to cure mental illness.* Harvard University Press.

Shorter, E. (2015). The history of nosology and the rise of the diagnostic and statistical manual of mental disorders. *Dialogues in Clinical Neuroscience, 17,* 59–67.

Spitzer, R. L., & Endicott, J. (1968). DIAGNO: A computer program for psychiatric diagnosis utilizing the differential diagnostic procedure. *Archives of General Psychiatry, 18,* 746–756.

Srole, L., Langner, T. S., Michael, S. T., Opler, M. K., & Rennie, T. A. C. (1962). *Mental health in the Metropolis: The midtown Manhattan study.* McGraw-Hill.

Starcevic, V., & Khazaal, Y. (2020). Problematic gaming, personality, and psychiatric disorders. *Frontiers in Psychiatry, 10,* 1004.

Stavropoulos, V., Gomez, R., & Motti-Stefanidi, F. (2019). Internet gaming disorder: A pathway towards assessment consensus. *Frontiers in Psychology, 10,* 1822.

Steel, Z., Marnane, C., Iranpour, C., Chey, T., Jackson, J., Patel, V., & Silove, D. (2014). The global prevalence of common mental disorders: A systematic review and meta-analysis 1980–2013. *International Journal of Epidemiology, 43,* 476–493.

Stier, M. (2013). Normative preconditions for the assessment of mental disorder. *Frontiers in Psychology, 4,* 611.

Sussman, S., Lisha, N., & Griffiths, M. (2011). Prevalence of the addictions: A problem of the majority or the minority? *Evaluation & the Health Professions, 34,* 3–56.

Tebartz van Elst, L. H. (2021). *Vom Anfang und Ende der Schizophrenie: Eine neuropsychiatrische Perspektive auf das Schizophrenie-Konzept.* Kohlhammer Verlag.

Thomas, R., Sanders, S., Doust, J., Beller, E., & Glasziou, P. (2015). Prevalence of attention-deficit/hyperactivity disorder: A systematic review and meta-analysis. *Pediatrics, 135,* e994–e1001.

Valenstein, E. S. (1974). *Brain control.* Wiley.

Van der Kolk, B. A. (2014). *The body keeps the score: Brain, mind, and body in the healing of trauma.* Viking.

Van Os, J. (2016). "Schizophrenia" does not exist. *BMJ. British Medical Journal, 352,* 1–2.

Van Os, J., & Linscott, R. J. (2012). Introduction: The extended psychosis phenotype—Relationship with schizophrenia and with ultrahigh risk status for psychosis. *Schizophrenia Bulletin, 38*, 227–230.

Varela, F. J., Thompson, E., & Rosch, E. (2017). *The embodied mind, revised edition: Cognitive science and human experience.* MIT Press.

Walters, J. (1998). Invading the Roman body: Manliness and impenetrability in Roman thought. In J. P. Hallett & M. B. Skinner (Eds.), *Roman sexualities* (pp. 29–43). Princeton University Press.

Watters, E. (2010). *Crazy like us: The globalization of the American psyche.* Free Press.

Willoughby, C. D. (2018). Running away from drapetomania: Samuel a. Cartwright, medicine, and race in the antebellum south. *Journal of Southern History, 84*, 579–614.

Wittchen, H. U., Jacobi, F., Rehm, J., Gustavsson, A., Svensson, M., Jonsson, B., Olesen, J., Allgulander, C., Alonso, J., Faravelli, C., Fratiglioni, L., & Steinhausen, H. C. (2011). The size and burden of mental disorders and other disorders of the brain in Europe 2010. *European Neuropsychopharmacology, 21*, 655–679.

Zachar, P., First, M. B., & Kendler, K. S. (2017). The bereavement exclusion debate in the DSM-5: A history. *Clinical Psychological Science, 5*, 890–906.

Zachar, P., & Kendler, K. S. (2012). The removal of Pluto from the class of planets and homosexuality from the class of psychiatric disorders: A comparison. *Philosophy, Ethics, and Humanities in Medicine, 7*, 1–7.

Zilles, K., & Amunts, K. (2010). Centenary of Brodmann's map—Conception and fate. *Nature Reviews Neuroscience, 11*, 139–145.

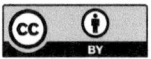

CHAPTER 3

Mental Enhancement

*Countries must learn how to capitalize on their citizens' cognitive
resources if they are to prosper, both economically and socially. Early
interventions will be key. To prosper and flourish in a rapidly changing
world, we must make the most of all our resources—both mental and
material. Globalization and its associated demands for competitiveness
are increasing the pressures in our working lives.*
—John R. Beddington, *then chief scientific adviser of the UK
government, and colleagues (Beddington et al., 2008, p. 1057)*

Abstract This chapter explains how people's nonmedical substance use,
particularly that of prescription stimulants, was understood as "enhancement" or "brain doping" since the early 2000s. In both the academic
debate and popular media, it was frequently claimed that ever more people, in particular students, were using such drugs to increase their cognitive performance. This chapter illustrates that this was not a new
phenomenon and that even "moral enhancement", the idea to use substances, and neuroscientific technology to improve people's moral behavior already existed in the 1960s and 1970s. The actual present prevalence
of brain doping is then discussed in detail, with an emphasis on other
motives to use drugs besides cognitive enhancement. Indeed, much of the
use turns out to be rather emotionally motivated and to cope with stress,
particularly in competitive environments, or to be even self-medication of
psychological problems. This shows how difficultly the distinction between

© The Author(s) 2023
S. Schleim, *Mental Health and Enhancement,* Palgrave Studies in
Law, Neuroscience, and Human Behavior,
https://doi.org/10.1007/978-3-031-32618-9_3

medical and nonmedical use can be drawn. Finally, nonpharmacological alternatives to improve one's mental health are presented. The chapter concludes that the academic debate on cognitive enhancement was not very informative and that a general theoretical framework for people's instrumental substance use should be preferred, which is introduced in Chap. 4.

Keywords Cognitive enhancement • Neuroenhancement • Moral enhancement • Coping • Stress • Science communication • Mental health

This quote is from the introduction to the article "The mental wealth of nations", which summarized the "Mental Capital and Wellbeing: Making the most of ourselves in the 21st century" research project, funded by the Government Office for Science of the UK and using a huge image of a brain on the cover of its report. The title obviously alludes to Adam Smith's (1723–1790) famous work, *The Wealth of Nations*, in which the Scottish economist and philosopher wrote about the generation of wealth through industrialization and free markets. The article's first author, John R. Beddington, is emeritus professor of biology and was the UK government's chief scientific adviser from 2008 until 2013. This emphasizes the significance of a project on "mental capital", which should also be seen in the context of deindustrialization in many developed countries, often poor in raw materials and thus reliant on intellectual work and property.

The quote is also a lesson in framing: Processes such as competition and globalization are described as inevitable facts, almost like a natural law, and the only way to "prosper and flourish" seems to be adaptation by maximizing performance. While it is difficult to measure psychological stress and whether it is increasing because we must essentially rely on subjective evaluations, we have here a group of leading experts testifying to "increasing pressures" in our lives. And, as we will see below, this report was carried out and completed during a time in which the enhancement debate gathered momentum in academia as well as in the media. The cultural background to the discussion that follows in this chapter is thus that of a competitive performance society. Although it is difficult to prove such complex interactions, we will actually find many links between performance pressure on the one hand and enhancement on the other. This is important insofar as it provides an alternative narrative: One of adapting to external pressure and coping with stress, compared to an intrinsic wish to improve oneself in a certain domain.

Here, we will not discuss in detail whether the situation is really as inevitable as the report stated. However, it is interesting to note that two years after the coronavirus pandemic, processes of deglobalization are also increasing in speed, as COVID-19 and the measures to prevent it exposed the dependence and vulnerability of a globalized economy in an unprecedented way. Related questions about the values underlying adaptive behavior will be addressed thoroughly at the end of Chap. 4 and in the final conclusion (Chap. 5). But in the context of the plea to improve people by the scientists and officials behind "Making the most of ourselves in the 21st century", one critical remark is helpful here: Imagine that you agreed with their conclusion that performance enhancement should be mandatory and there were relatively safe means—more on that later—to raise your IQ from 100 to 110. After "improving" yourself accordingly, the question whether this higher level of intelligence was sufficient or whether performance should be increased further would arise again. Also imagine the competitive pressure due to others, nationally as well as globally, making use of similar means.

So, once we take that road, it quickly becomes a slippery slope. Whether we aim for an IQ of 120, 130, 140, or even higher, the demand for further improvement would always arise again. (We acknowledge here that "higher IQ" does not always translate into better functioning. It is just meant as a simple illustration.) Also imagine that making use of these means comes at a cost, financially as well as the time and effort spent, and with the risk of side effects. It is thus very likely that performance enhancement in an already-competitive and stressful environment will, at least in the long run, only lead to reiterations of these aspects at continuously higher levels, both of benefits and of costs.

A visual illustration of this critical conclusion is presented in the report's own summary, although this was probably unintended by the authors. "The mental wealth of nations" includes a figure showing positive and negative influences on people's "mental capital". Enhancement already begins before birth ("fetal programming") and then continues throughout life. The notion that people get older and retire from work is literally called a "waste of mental capital" (Beddington et al., 2008, p. 1059).

Drugs and alcohol, relevant to our topic, are mentioned as a negative influence, alongside childhood trauma and social isolation. The most prominent negative factor is stress. While this may already sound complex, it is actually only the simple picture as published in *Nature*. To see the scientists' original figure, one has to download a more complicated version.[1] This combines so many factors that parents, as well as people of all ages, must consider that the endeavor to "boost brain power in young and old" and prevent negative influences could be quite exhausting. In fact, such intensive efforts to increase a nation's "mental capital" might themselves stress people out—which would have negative effects according to the proposal itself and thus run counter to the whole project.

The above should suffice to exemplify the complexity of mental or cognitive enhancement, both on the individual and on the global level, at the outset of this chapter. In what follows, we will summarize the scholarly debate and its representation in the media, answer the question about prevalence, and discuss nonpharmacological forms of enhancement. As mentioned, the substances used will be addressed in more detail in Chap. 4.

3.1   THE DEBATE

As the "Decade of the Brain" approached its end in 2000, scholars from different disciplines, such as neuroscience, law, and philosophy, increasingly identified ethical issues related to brain research. Some found it necessary to address them in new disciplines such as "neuroethics" or "neurolaw" (Schleim, 2020a). How meaningful this nomenclature is will not concern us here any further, but the proliferation of ever more "neuro" terms has provoked critique by some (De Vries, 2007; Vidal & Piperberg, 2017; Wilfond & Ravitsky, 2005). As a matter of fact, ethical issues about the brain, neurology, and psychiatry were being discussed long before some researchers coined the new terminology. Examples in medical ethics or bioethics are legion and can already be found in the context of brain stimulation and psychosurgery in the 1950s through to the 1970s (Schleim, 2021; Valenstein, 1974).

In particular, one of the topics that has received increasing attention since the early 2000s is cognitive or neuroenhancement (Fig. 3.1). The

---

[1] "The mental wealth of nations", online at: https://www.nature.com/articles/4551057a

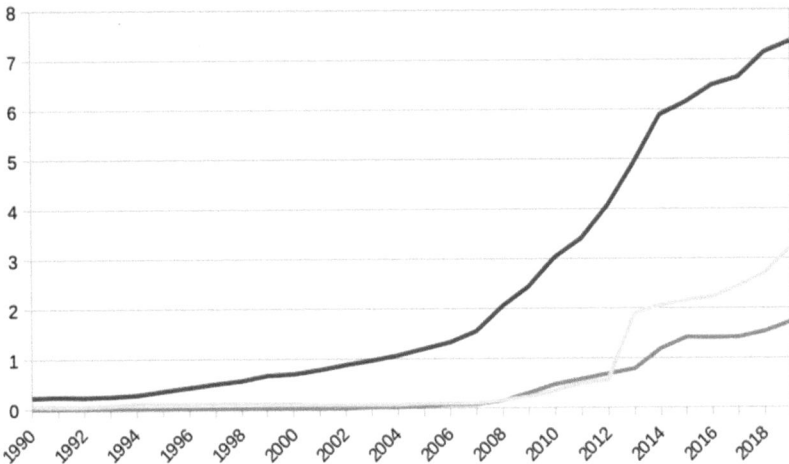

Fig. 3.1 Increasing Attention to Cognitive Enhancement. Cognitive enhancement is increasingly addressed in English-language books from the 1990s (blue line). Neuroenhancement is a less common term, although its use has also been increasing in recent years (red line). Moral enhancement (yellow line) has gained increasing attention since a seminal publication in 2008. (Source: Google Ngram (lines smoothed; ×10^8))

same pattern can also be found in academic journals (Schleim & Quednow, 2017). Furthermore, O'Connor and colleagues have shown that the topic of enhancing and optimizing the brain even dominated media coverage of neuroscience, with 43.4% of the articles addressing the subject (O'Connor et al., 2012). There is thus ample evidence from different sources that the topic of this chapter played and still plays a major role in discourses about the brain and applications of neuroscience.

We have already discussed the common definition of "enhancement" in the introduction, even reflected in the title *Beyond Therapy* chosen by the US President's Council on Bioethics (President's Council on Bioethics, 2003). In spite of the definition's tentative and pragmatic character already being acknowledged 20 years ago, it is still guiding research on the topic. For example, in a recent review of open questions in the debate, Racine and colleagues characterized cognitive enhancement as "the use of medications or other brain treatments for improving normal healthy cognition" (Racine et al., 2021, p. 2, quoting Farah, 2015). In the introduction to a new special issue on the topic, Hope and colleagues similarly referred to the understanding of enhancement common among ethicists, as "interventions that are used to improve human form or functioning beyond what is necessary to restore or sustain health" (Hope et al., 2021, p.1, quoting Juengst & Moseley, 2019). Racine and colleagues' definition is more narrow in that it only refers to "cognition" and limits the means to "medications or brain treatments", while Juengst and Mosley's broadly speaks of "interventions"—and actually also includes body image. However, both definitions share the "beyond therapy" idea: Enhancement means *improvement beyond healthy or normal functioning*. Cognitive or moral neuroenhancement—what does that precisely mean? We have not yet addressed these concepts in detail. Let us begin with a brief reflection on the latter.

Moral Enhancement

After what has now become a seminal and highly cited paper by moral philosopher Thomas Douglas from the University of Oxford, who argued that this kind of improvement is ethically permissible, ever more neuroscientists, psychologists, and philosophers have taken up the idea. Douglas presented a rather pessimistic view of people when he wrote:

> There is clearly scope for most people to morally enhance themselves. According to every plausible moral theory, people often have bad or suboptimally good motives. And according to many plausible theories, some of the world's most important problems—such as developing world poverty, climate change and war—can be attributed to these moral deficits. (Douglas, 2008, p. 230)

The philosopher presupposed that "biomedical moral enhancement technologies will become technically feasible in the medium term future" (ibid., p. 242). According to his view, people's moral behavior could be improved by changing their emotions in such a way that they give rise to better motives, which then lead to better actions. In the subsequent debate, this was often understood as pharmacologically instigating prosocial or altruistic emotions (see also Langlitz et al., 2021; Schleim, 2011; 2022a). Note how weak Douglas's original point actually was, arguing only for the permissibility of moral enhancement if people choose this for themselves. However, if people, in general, really have such bad motives, as he assumed, why should they themselves make the choice in the first place? And would not other means be available to improve their actions, such as moral education? Changing their emotion, by contrast, without their informed consent, would be a serious violation of their autonomy and resemble a totalitarian doctrine.

In addition to this ethical problem, moral enhancement obviously raises questions about the feasibility of such a project. While the debate has not only been ongoing but actually growing for many years (Fig. 3.1), there is still no clarity about how moral enhancement should be applied in practice. Douglas's hope for a solution to be available "in the medium term future" is relativized when one realizes what has been overlooked in neuroethics thus far—that moral enhancement was already proposed in the 1960s and 1970s. For example, brain researcher José M. R. Delgado (1915–2011) wanted to "psychocivilize" the entire population by implanting remote-controlled brain reading and stimulating devices, which he called "stimoceivers" (Delgado, 1971; Schleim, 2021). The device was developed in animals and later tested in some humans as well, particularly psychiatric patients.

For Delgado, its application would be mandatory to prevent humankind from destroying itself, which can be understood better in the context of the Cold War (1945–1990). As the brain researcher was convinced that his method would first be developed and applied to treat patients with mental disorders, thus having the opportunity to refine it and improve its safety, he perceived the realization of his vision merely as a question of time and found the ethical issues manageable. However, several years later, he relativized his views on the potential of neurotechnology and promoted its use in combination with the improvement of social structures and education to help people better control themselves (Delgado, 1983; Fins & Vernaglia, 2022). This change of mind occurred after he lost funding for his neuroscientific vision, as he failed to convince other scientists and important decision-makers that his brain stimulation devices could indeed be used to control animals' or people's emotions (see Snyder, 2009).

The idea of improving people scientifically was widespread during this period, even if scholars were not yet calling it "moral enhancement" (see also Somit, 1976). Behaviorist Burrhus F. Skinner (1904–1990), for example, wanted to change the reward structure of the environment such that people would behave better (Skinner, 1971). He called his method "cultural design" and was widely criticized for promoting a totalitarian idea. In the same year, *TIME Magazine* published a report entitled "A Pill for Peace?" and quoted from a speech of Kenneth Clark (1914–2005), then president of the American Psychological Association (APA), at an APA meeting in Washington, DC. According to the report, the psychologist stated that "[t]he world's leaders [...] should be required to take 'psychotechnological medication'—pills or other treatments to curb their aggressive behavior and induce them to govern more humanely."[2] The journalist writing about Clark's speech found this "an extraordinarily dramatic extension" of Skinner's approach and view "that man must be controlled to survive." The report also addressed the dilemma, mentioned above, concerning informed consent, which has thus not been resolved more than 50 years later:

> How possibly could the drug dispensers differentiate between the power drive that constitutes leadership and that which leads to aggressive violence? And who would dispense the drugs? If they were voluntary, those most in need of them would be precisely those who would not take them. If they could somehow be made obligatory, then the dispensers would become the dominators. Who polices the police?[3]

So much for moral enhancement, which was already promoted by scientists decades before the "Decade of the Brain" and the advent of neuroethics. This example vividly illustrates not only the complexity of tinkering with the brain, but also the obliviousness of present ethical debates to the historical dimension. As we will see shortly, this is unfortunately not the only example in this respect. Let us now have a closer look at cognitive or neuroenhancement, which has received the most attention in science and the media to date.

Cognitive or Neuroenhancement

"Cognition" is in itself a broad term, encompassing perception, thought processes, and decision-making. It is often used as the counterpart to "emotion", but sometimes also in a broader sense to denote psychological processes as a whole, as in "cognitive science" (Greene et al., 2004). We will use it here in the former, more narrow, sense. To understand a little

---

[2] "A Pill for Peace?", *TIME Magazine* of September 20, 1971, Vol. 98, Issue 12, p.10.
[3] Ibid.

better what cognitive enhancement is about, we will look at a few experimental studies investigating the effects of certain drugs on healthy people.

One particularly illustrative example is an investigation of the effects of methylphenidate—better known under the brand name Ritalin—on cognitive ability and decision-making by Agay et al. (2010). Although their primary interest was the drug's effect on subjects with an ADHD diagnosis, they also had a healthy control group, as well as a placebo condition for both groups. Interestingly enough, the three different psychological tasks they used yielded three different outcomes: For the first test, the "digit-span task", participants were shown increasingly longer sequences of digits for a short period of time, which they then had to reproduce either forwards or backwards. The healthy subjects receiving methylphenidate correctly remembered about 65% of the digits, compared to roughly 60% in the placebo group (Agay et al., 2010).[4]

The second task was about decision-making to maximize financial rewards and minimize losses. In the "Iowa Gambling Task", subjects draw cards from four decks with different reward/loss structures. The challenge is to find out which of them, in the long run, yield the highest benefits. This was originally developed by neurologists in Iowa to investigate functional deficits in patients with a particular kind of frontal lobe brain damage. However, methylphenidate did not affect the outcomes between the groups for this part of the experiment (nor for the subjects with an ADHD diagnosis).

For the third condition, the researchers developed an alternative version of the previous task which they called "Foregone Payoff Gambling Task". In addition to the card decks having a different reward/loss structure, for each card chosen the participants also saw what the results would have been for the other decks, thus what their "foregone payoffs" were. This made the task cognitively more demanding. Surprisingly, the subjects without an ADHD diagnosis who were given the drug made more disadvantageous choices than those in the placebo group—slightly above 30% compared to slightly below 25%—and thus had a worse outcome (Agay et al., 2010).

---

[4] This study is discussed here to illustrate the complexity of investigating cognitive enhancement. To avoid making the description overly complex, I only refer here to descriptive statistics and omit the discussion of statistical significance. As is common in this kind of research, the sample size—16 per condition in the non-ADHD group and 13 per condition in the ADHD group—is too small to allow conclusions about the general population.

We can draw three important conclusions from this brief summary of the study. Firstly, researchers often use laboratory tests designed to measure performance differences in clinical populations. It is unclear what the results from such tasks—remembering digits or drawing cards—mean for people's everyday lives. We must thus be aware of what I have previously called a "translational fallacy" (Schleim, 2014a), consisting in the premature translation of clinical tests into real life. Secondly, we should not expect too much of the substances used. This single study is obviously too limited to draw general conclusions, but the effects of substance use that we have seen here are rather modest and probably practically irrelevant, even *if* the tasks could easily be translated into people's everyday lives. Thirdly, the results are also inconsistent, because they suggest an improvement in some domains, no performance difference in others, and even an impairment in yet other conditions. Pharmacologists have previously emphasized that the cognitive effects of drugs can be quite complex, with a gain in one domain potentially accompanied by an impairment in another. There is, in particular, no "more is better" guarantee, but rather an optimal level of functioning, above which an improvement can become an impairment (see Quednow, 2010).

Is there, then, no more conclusive evidence? Considering the caveats discussed above, one exceptional study examined 39 healthy male chess players with an average age of 37.3 years (Franke et al., 2017). They were asked to play several games against a chess computer adapted to their level of performance to keep the difficulty similar for all participants. The substances administered were, again, methylphenidate, or modafinil (Provigil), a drug primarily prescribed for particular sleeping disorders, as well as caffeine, or a placebo. To obtain as much meaningful data as possible from a still relatively small group of subjects, all players participated over four days. At each visit, they received a different substance, without of course knowing which. The playing time per game was limited to 15 minutes.

On average, the chess players scored 6.3% (methylphenidate) to 8.2% (modafinil) more points per game compared to the placebo. However, these increases were too small to reach the statistical significance threshold. The performance differences between the caffeine and methylphenidate consumption groups were negligible. Compared to the freely available caffeine, the chess players scored an average of 1.7% more points under the influence of the prescription drug modafinil, but this difference was also not statistically significant. Surprisingly, chess players took more time per game after administration of any of the two medical drugs and therefore lost more often because they ran out of time. The researchers speculated that the participants would have performed better under the influence of the active substances if there had been no time limit (Franke et al., 2017). This study is remarkable in that it was carried out under relatively realistic conditions—at least for chess players. In this sense, the first of the three caveats—addressing the "translational fallacy"—is met. It would still require further research, though, to generalize this to other applied contexts. The second caveat, that the effects in such studies are usually small, was confirmed by the chess players' data. Without going into the details of the meaning of "statistical significance" and its relation to practical relevance, it should be obvious that such substances will not make a chess master out of a beginner. However, they could still be useful: In very competitive situations, such as professional sports, where the performance of all participants is similar due to preselection, even a small difference of 1.7% *can* mean a lot. Modafinil is actually considered a doping substance in sports and its use in combination with medical problems has repeatedly sparked debate (see Kaufman, 2005). The substance is thus also banned from certain chess tournaments, unless a participant has a valid exemption. However, the third caveat, emphasizing possible trade-offs of substance use, was also reaffirmed by the chess study, with the players, on average, making better decisions, but at the cost of time.

In contrast to the popular but also vague notion of "smart drugs", we have now gained a preliminary understanding of what cognitive enhancement means in research and how it is investigated. In more psychological terms, we might keep in mind that such experimental tasks investigate processes such as attention, working memory, planning, and decision-making. We will draw a firmer conclusion on the effects of these substances in healthy people in the chapter on substances. Also note that the focus of that chapter will be on stimulant drugs, as they are the most frequently used substances in the context of neuroenhancement. For the aims of this section, we will now summarize the central arguments in the debate before discussing the prevalence question in the subsequent section.

Central Arguments

The annual number of papers on cognitive or neuroenhancement on the *Web of Science*, a common database for scientific publications, already exceeded 100 in 2013 (Schleim & Quednow, 2017). It is now approaching 200 and that database alone presently lists 2086 entries on the topic. However, the *Web of Science* does not cover all scientific journals, and, in particular, it does not list books or book chapters, in which academics also disseminate and discuss their research. These figures should make it clear that we cannot summarize the whole debate here, but we also need not do so. In the following paragraphs, we will address a couple of very influential or very recent publications.

A highly cited and influential review coauthored by, among others, Nobel laureate and neurologist Eric Kandel, as well as the influential British neuropsychologist Barbara Sahakian, professor at the University of Cambridge and one of the authors of "The mental wealth of nations" (Beddington et al., 2008), was published in 2004 in *Nature Reviews Neuroscience* (Farah et al., 2004). These authors claimed that "[o]ur growing ability to alter brain function can be used to enhance the mental processes of normal individuals" (ibid., p. 421). They pointed out that in some school districts in the US prescription stimulants (such as methylphenidate or amphetamine) were consumed at a rate that could not solely be understood on the basis of ADHD diagnoses, for which these drugs are commonly prescribed. There was, furthermore, evidence that on some campuses as many as 16% of students might take these substances. Nutritional supplements promising improved memory were also gaining in popularity. The authors concluded from this that "pharmacological enhancement has already begun" (ibid., p. 421). They later wrote about "the advent of widespread neurocognitive enhancement" (ibid., p. 422) and then briefly addressed the ethical issues of safety, coercion, distributive justice, and personhood, before stating that "[n]eurocognitive enhancement is already a fact of life for many people" (ibid., p. 424). They also called for an interdisciplinary discussion involving neuroscientists as well as ethicists, and then concluded:

> With many of our college students already using stimulants to enhance executive function and the pharmaceutical industry soon to be offering an array of new memory-enhancing drugs, the time to begin this discussion is now. (ibid., p. 424)

A few years later, some of the coauthors of that article published another highly cited article, this time in *Nature*, with Henry Greely, professor of law at Stanford University, as first author (Greely et al., 2008). "Towards responsible use of cognitive-enhancing drugs by the healthy", the title of that article, can be understood as an academic manifesto in favor of the practice. It started out with the claim that "[s]ociety must respond to the growing demand for cognitive enhancement" (ibid., p. 702), followed by the statement that students are using substances such as amphetamine or methylphenidate "not to get high, but to get higher grades, to provide an edge over their fellow students" (ibid.). The authors then referred to research suggesting that "almost 7% of students in US universities have used prescription stimulants in this way, and that on some campuses, up to 25% of students had used them in the past year" (ibid.). They also addressed issues of safety, coercion, and fairness. Responsible use of the drugs for them consisted in maximizing benefits while minimizing harm, expressed in seven demands (Box 3.1). Greely and colleagues eventually concluded:

> We should welcome new methods of improving our brain function. In a world in which human work-spans and lifespans are increasing, cognitive enhancement tools—including the pharmacological—will be increasingly useful for improved quality of life and extended work productivity [...]. (Greely et al., 2008, p. 705)

Box 3.1   Seven Demands for Cognitive Enhancement

In the manifesto, "Towards responsible use", Greely and colleagues called for

- a presumption that mentally competent adults should be able to engage in cognitive enhancement by using drugs;
- an evidence-based approach to the evaluation of the risks and benefits of cognitive enhancement;
- enforceable policies concerning the use of cognitive-enhancing drugs to support fairness, protect individuals from coercion, and minimize enhancement-related socioeconomic disparities;
- a program of research into the use and impacts of cognitive-enhancing drugs by healthy individuals;
- physicians, educators, regulators, and others to collaborate in developing policies that address the use of cognitive-enhancing drugs by healthy individuals;
- information to be broadly disseminated concerning the risks, benefits, and alternatives to pharmaceutical enhancement; and
- careful and limited legislative action to channel cognitive enhancement technologies into useful paths.

The next two sources were published between what I called the "manifesto" and the present. In 2013, the specialized journal, *Neuropharmacology*, hosted a debate on cognitive enhancement between three renowned scientists. This journal primarily addresses a certain branch of science, unlike the much broader *Nature* journals mentioned above. The three participants were Steve E. Hyman, who at that time held a professorship at Harvard University and had previously been Thomas Insel's predecessor at the US National Institute of Mental Health; Nora D. Volkow, director of the US National Institute on Drug Abuse; and David Nutt, professor of neuropsychopharmacology at Imperial College London (Hyman et al., 2013).

Nutt took a very positive stance on enhancement, referring to stimulant use in the military and describing it as a logical follow-up to biological evolution. Hyman took a moderately positive position, but also highlighted the problems of fairness and coercion, particularly in competitive settings. Volkow pointed out that, in the US, 8% of 12th graders had used amphetamine nonmedically in the previous year and that the stimulant is known for its addictive potential. She also called it a "fairy tale" that there will be a "magic bullet" or "a medication that will improve all of a sudden our cognitive abilities" (ibid., p. 10). Volkow, furthermore, voiced doubts that unless healthy people are sleep deprived, stimulant drugs actually improve their cognition.

With similar critical thoughts, Martha Farah, a cognitive neuroscientist, professor at the University of Pennsylvania, and active in neuroethics since its very inception, published the essay "The unknowns of cognitive enhancement" in *Science* (Farah, 2015). This is particularly remarkable, as she also coauthored the two enthusiastic articles in the *Nature* journals mentioned above. In comparison to the "manifesto", her thoughtful piece received much less attention—not even 8% of the citations on *Google Scholar*, for example. This may be only circumstantial evidence that the present communication culture pays much more attention to optimistic rather than neutral or even critical content, but is corroborated by more systematic analyses (see Partridge et al., 2011; Racine et al., 2010).

Farah referred to new research questioning the enhancing effects of stimulant drugs in healthy subjects, raised the problem of dependence, and then illustrated an aspect of the experiments already familiar to us: "As with amphetamine, studies have produced conflicting results. A recent literature review of the cognitive effects of modafinil found a range of outcomes: enhancement, null effects, and occasionally impairment" (Farah,

2015, p. 380, referring to Battleday & Brem, 2015). To be fair to the evidence, most studies reported positive (i.e., enhancing) results—but this must be seen in the context of the now widely known publication bias, that is, the fact that most scientific journals reject null findings. Farah concludes: "Given that enhancements would likely be used for years, long-term effectiveness and safety are essential concerns but are particularly difficult and costly to determine" (ibid., p. 380). Barbara Sahakian and a collaborator had pointed out the importance of understanding long-term effects in a similar fashion almost ten years earlier:

> Despite the difficulties inherent in monitoring the effects of drug usage over several years, a full exploration of the long-term implications of new treatments is vital, especially those that might routinely be used by the healthy population. (Turner & Sahakian, 2006, p. 82)

The final two reviews I want to address here have in common that they try to summarize and systematize almost 20 years of the neuroenhancement debate. They were both published in specialized journals and by authors from a younger generation of researchers. In "Hacking the Brain: Dimensions of Cognitive Enhancement", Martin Dresler and colleagues distinguish seven dimensions and three strategies of cognitive enhancement (Dresler et al., 2019). The strategies are the means, namely behavioral (e.g., sleep, meditation, and computer training), biochemical (e.g., nutrition and pharmaceuticals), and physical (e.g., gadgets, implants, and electrical stimulation). The dimensions are the perspectives from which one can look at the strategies, such as the cognitive domain to be improved (e.g., memory, creativity, and attention), personal factors interacting with the means (e.g., intelligence, age, and genes), and side effects. The authors conclude that "[c]ognitive enhancement clearly is a multidimensional endeavor" calling for "a more differentiated approach" (ibid., pp. 1142–1143). Put differently, all the means and dimensions potentially matter and have to be considered in further research. We will come back to this in the chapter's conclusion.

Most recently, Racine and colleagues identified and discussed "Unanswered Questions About Human Psychology and Social Behavior" regarding cognitive enhancement (Racine et al., 2021), identifying important "gaps" in the ethical discussion to date, thus over roughly 20 years of scholarly activity. They formulate three major questions that should be addressed in further research. Firstly, which psychological and social outcomes should be enhanced? Secondly, what are the similarities and differences between the various methods (i.e., what the previous group of authors called "strategies") of enhancement? And thirdly, what are the motivations of people to engage in cognitive enhancement?

The first question is remarkable in that it raises the fundamental concern of the whole debate. We have seen above that "cognition" is a very broad term and that researchers use a variety of experimental designs to measure it. What I find so remarkable is that one might expect more clarity on so basic a question after two decades of debate. However, the review discussed above also took the pragmatic approach of listing more or less everything that could be included in the "cognitive domain" (Dresler et al., 2019).

With their second major question, Racine and colleagues stress how important it is to carry out research in real-life settings, which we also addressed as a caveat above. The authors discuss much more complexity and finally conclude:

> The growth of biotechnology and neuroscience yields numerous possibilities for the development of cognitive enhancement. [...] Extensive research into these aspects is imperative if we are to assess the ethics of the (non-)use of cognitive enhancers in an evidence-based and integrative manner and inform future policy making as well as technology development. (Racine et al., 2021, pp. 18–19)

This sounds as if the research were just about to begin—but as we have seen above, there are already more than 2000 related publications listed on the *Web of Science* alone. If the debate has been unable to yield any more clarity in 20 years, can we be sure of substantial improvement after another 20 years? We will also keep this conclusion in mind for the end of the chapter. However, before getting there, we will actually question two other foundational aspects of the neuroenhancement debate that have not yet been addressed: What is it that people change when they take the common substances? And how prevalent is that behavior?

Is it Really About Cognition?

Attentive readers might find some of the messages communicated thus far paradoxical, if not contradictory: On the one hand, many scholars have stated or at least suggested that cognitive enhancement is common and increasing. Yet, on the other hand, experimental studies of what the drugs—in particular, prescription stimulants—are actually doing to their users have yielded ambiguous results. Meanwhile, there have been many such attempts, sometimes in the context of clinical research involving healthy control groups, as with the first study we discussed above (Agay et al., 2010), and sometimes specifically with healthy people, to directly investigate the potential of cognitive enhancement in that group, as with the chess players (Franke et al., 2017).

To put the paradox in a provocative way: Why would so many normally functioning people pay for and use the drugs, risking and in some cases actually suffering from side effects, if the substances are doing nothing? *Why are the users using, if that's of no use?* Or could it be that the experimental researchers are not investigating the effects correctly? Does cognition need to be measured differently or do the drugs affect something else instead? So, who is wrong here, the scientists or the users? A plausible answer is inspired by another researcher.

In an article published in 2013, the sociologist Scott Vrecko of King's College in London did something nobody else in the field of neuroethics had done before: He actually interviewed users of so-called cognitive enhancers to learn more about their motives (Vrecko, 2013). While quantitative research employs strict standardization in large samples of people to generalize findings to the whole population (and, in reality, many researchers only investigate their medical or psychology students out of convenience), Vrecko took a qualitative approach: He used semi-structured interviews—basically a number of prepared questions defining the focus of interest, while allowing the interviewees to answer freely—to talk to 24 students "attending an elite university on the East Coast of the United States" (ibid., p. 5). His results thus cannot be generalized to all users at all locations, but this is also not necessary to inform the debate. What the students told him was both remarkably consistent and remarkably different from the way the phenomenon had thus far been described in the scholarly debate.

According to the recruitment procedure, the interviewees needed to have experience with prescription stimulants as a study aid but did not consider themselves to have ADHD or a similar diagnosis. None of them apparently wanted to become the "next little Einstein". Instead, they described their stimulant use in ways that led Vrecko to identify the following four motives: (1) feeling up, (2) drivenness, (3) interestedness, and (4) enjoyment. The first reflects an increased level of energy and well-being, and the second a strong desire to do something. To illustrate the latter, one student said that under the influence of the drug (containing amphetamine) she would "just sit down and do whatever it is I have to do and won't feel okay until I finish it" (ibid., p. 8). The third category concerned students finding their academic work more interesting and the fourth that they enjoyed it more. The answer to the question Vrecko formulated as, "Just How Cognitive Is 'Cognitive Enhancement'?", also his article's title, thus seems to be: What academics have commonly described as cognitive enhancement, instead appears to be about *emotion and motivation*.

When I present these findings in my lectures and seminars about the performance society, I usually tell my students that if they need drugs to find my teaching interesting enough to pay attention, I might better be replaced by another professor. I only half mean this as a joke: Results such as Vrecko's indicate that students have insufficient intrinsic motivation to do what they are supposed to do. Again, it must be stressed that this conclusion is not representative of academia at large. Perhaps these students chose the wrong program to study. To a certain extent, it is also normal that we, whether at school, at work, or anywhere else, are not always so absorbed by what we are doing that time flies and we feel a sense of flow.

What I want to point out here is the possibility that the students' lack of emotional connection with and motivation for what they are doing could also tell us something about their academic environment. Magon Inon, then a researcher in education at University College London, similarly suggested taking students' emotions seriously, as a meaningful response to the reality they live in (Inon, 2019). It is important to stress that individual adaptation by changing emotion is not the only option in such a situation. The environment could also be adapted to the individuals' needs—or individuals could move to surroundings better matching their own possibilities and needs. We neither can nor need to comprehensively resolve this issue here. For our purpose, it matters primarily that "cognitive enhancement", in spite of its high prevalence in the literature (Fig. 3.1), does not seem to be the appropriate description of the phenomenon, at least in some scientifically documented cases. I thus prefer the term "neuroenhancement" and will opt to even drop that nomenclature at the end of the chapter.

Vrecko's results are not the only ones suggesting such an alternative understanding of the phenomenon. A few years later, British researchers undertook a similar study at a university in England (Vargo & Petróczi,

2016). Unfortunately, their sample (eight habitual and five sporadic users) was even smaller than that of the previous study. However, this in itself is an interesting fact: They started out with five students who they knew— from earlier research and their own social network—were engaged in neuroenhancement. These students were in turn asked to establish contact with other users. When they reached a total of 13, no further participants could be found. This clearly contradicts the notion of neuroenhancement being a mass phenomenon.

At first glance, these researchers seem to reinforce the idea of students using substances for performance enhancement: "Primarily, participants hoped neuroenhancement would help them to 'pull an all-nighter,' boost their concentration, energy and motivation toward the task at hand" (ibid., p. 5). However, the complete analysis of their interviews showed that the students' "motivations to neuroenhance resided in their need to 'catch up' and cope with their work related demands" (ibid., p. 8), particularly among lower achieving students. Consistent with earlier research showing that medical drugs containing amphetamine or methylphenidate are more difficult to obtain in the UK than in the US (Singh et al., 2014), the preferred substance of students was modafinil, with which we are already familiar from the chess study.

In conclusion, Vargo and Petróczi confirmed Vrecko's findings that neuroenhancement is mostly about emotion and motivation, especially coping with stress in competitive environments: "Neuroenhancement seems to be an adaptation to work-hard play-hard lifestyles, as well as to the competitiveness of contemporary higher education" (Vargo & Petróczi, 2016, p. 10). As previously, students' answers were remarkably consistent on that point. Remember that these qualitative findings from small samples are not the only evidence we have. We started out with the paradox that people are using prescription stimulants despite the results of experimental research on their cognitive effects being rather modest or ambiguous. This in itself calls for an alternative explanation, which the interview studies discussed here provide. These are, in turn, backed up by further surveys and experimental research that support the interpretation that the stimulant drugs primarily affect motivation—at least in healthy people who are not sleep deprived (see Ilieva & Farah, 2013, 2019; Müller et al., 2013).

Taken together, this evidence undermines the common narrative in neuroethics that "cognitive enhancement" is really about cognition or getting smarter, instead of coping with stress in a competitive environment or a lack of motivation, which we might simply call "boredom". This implies that the common notion of "smart drugs" might be entirely misleading (see also Elliott & Elliott, 2011; Inon, 2019). There will be more evidence in this respect in the next section, where we finally discuss quantitative research on the prevalence of neuroenhancement.

3.2   How Common is It Really?

In the seminal publications on neuroenhancement summarized above, we found statements claiming that up to 16% or even 25% of students were using stimulant drugs non-medically, at least on some campuses. This practice has also often been described as common and increasing. However, the evidence for both of these claims is less clear than one may think. Early in the debate, one of my later collaborators (Quednow, 2010) and I (Schleim, 2010) cautioned against the proliferation of such high numbers more broadly. Similarly, researchers at the University of Queensland in Australia identified a "neuroenhancement bubble" (Lucke et al., 2011) or investigated the media hype about it (Partridge et al., 2011). According to the latter study, 94% of such articles presented neuroenhancement as common, increasing, or both, and 95% described the benefits, compared to only 58% mentioning risks or side effects. Exaggerating the benefits and downplaying the risks might actually also be characteristic of the ethical debate and not just what journalists are doing (Heinz & Müller, 2017). But what precisely does the scientific evidence tell us about the prevalence of the phenomenon?[5]

This question was the subject of a comprehensive review of 28 individual studies as early as 2011 (Smith & Farah, 2011). However, the results ranged between 1.7% and 55%, with so much variability indicating inconsistent approaches among researchers. For example, how did they each define the phenomenon, and how did they subsequently measure it in practice? The research groups seem to have different answers to these questions. It is noteworthy that Smith and Farah also found that in some surveys the reported prevalence correlated with the competitiveness in that context.

---

[5] The following paragraphs of this section are adapted from my report on brain doping (Schleim, 2022b), which can be accessed online at: https://doi.org/10.33612/227882920

More recently, a new paper was published, which summarized 111 studies (Faraone et al., 2020). Their results varied even more—between 2.1% and 58.7%. These authors also regretted that, due to the different methodologies of the individual studies, they were unable to conduct a formal meta-analysis that would have allowed them to summarize the empirical findings in a standardized manner. The evidence base in 2020 has thus hardly improved since 2011. The honest answer to the prevalence question is, therefore, that we cannot really say with any certainty how many people engage in neuroenhancement. We can, however, reflect on what is plausible.

For example, the results of studies that are more methodologically sound, in which substantially more people (N > 10,000) were surveyed—ideally using a representative method and conducted at different locations—are usually in the single-digit percentage range. By contrast, the extreme value of 55% originated from a nonrepresentative survey of a few (n = 307) male members of fraternities at only one North American university (DeSantis et al., 2009). Young men and members of such fraternities are known for their excessive substance use. In contrast to this, the representative US National Survey on Drug Use and Health 2015–2016 (n = 102,000) found that only 2.1% of respondents had used prescription stimulants such as amphetamine or methylphenidate without a prescription (Compton et al., 2018). Furthermore, a large-scale, international comparative study reported that substance use is higher in English-speaking countries (e.g., Canada, the US, and the UK) than in German-speaking countries (Germany, Austria, and Switzerland; Maier et al., 2018). This indicates cultural differences in neuroenhancement.

Many of these studies, however, did not specifically focus on cognitive or neuroenhancement, but on the "non-medical use" of stimulants and other substances. This includes motivations such as wanting to party longer, wanting to overcome social anxiety or shyness, wanting to lose weight (some substances suppress hunger), or simply wanting to experience a "high". Yet, these crucial differences are often overlooked in many reports, both in scientific publications and in general media. Improved concentration or staying awake longer to study were also frequently mentioned as reasons for substance use. However, this could simply reflect the fact that most of the surveys were conducted among students. In their stage of life and situation, these are, after all, essential activities.

The evidence discussed in the previous section, furthermore, showed that the more "academic" reasons might refer to improving motivation or coping with stress rather than the genuine wish to become smarter. However, such nuances are difficult to consider in quantitative research, although they can, as we have seen above, substantially affect the interpretation of the results. Unsurprisingly, those studies that focus exclusively on enhancing academic performance rather than asking about "non-medical use", in general, report considerably lower frequency of use.

The clearest indication that there has been *any* increase in use at all is provided by researchers at the University of Michigan (McCabe et al., 2014). They repeated a nonrepresentative survey at the same university on six occasions between 2003 and 2013. This revealed an increase in non-medical use of prescription stimulants from 5.4% to 9.3% over that period. It is important to note that the survey participants were asked whether they had consumed stimulants *at least once in the last year*. This obviously does not tell us anything about the frequency of the use, which could be several times a day, a few times a week, or also just once in a whole year. Fortunately, the same research group examined this issue in a separate investigation (Teter et al., 2010). According to that study, 82.1% of the users had taken stimulants less than ten times in total. So, even though more students had tried such substances, around four out of five stopped using them after a few times. Apparently, they neither became dependent nor found the stimulant drugs very useful.

Comparison to the Past

These and many other findings strongly suggest that cognitive or neuroenhancement has never been a mass phenomenon and by no means can we say with any certainty that it has increased in the last 20 years. Contemporary figures may even be lower than those of surveys from the 1960s to the 1980s, which are summarized in more detail in previous publications (Schleim, 2020b; Schleim & Quednow, 2017, 2018). Similarly to the precursors of contemporary brain stimulation or moral enhancement, the neuroethics debate was oblivious to these empirical findings. But let us discuss here a few historical examples at least briefly.

One review paper covered 21 individual surveys from 1966 to 1980 (McAuliffe et al., 1984). In these, between 11% and 54% of the participants stated that they had previously taken amphetamines, mainly for the purpose of staying awake longer, to perform better on a test, or in sports. Note that methylphenidate was not well known at the time. Not long after, the same research group published a detailed but nonrepresentative survey of health science professionals and students (n = 1308; McAuliffe et al., 1986). Some 16% of the doctors and 17% of the medical students surveyed reported that they had taken drugs or medication to stay awake longer, to work more effectively, or to be better at sports. The professionals estimated that they had done so roughly 44 times on average; for the students, the figure was 66 times. This is significantly higher than the numbers presented by the researchers in 2010 (Teter et al., 2010). It is therefore entirely conceivable that cognitive or neuroenhancement was even more widespread in the past than it is today, even if people did not yet call it that.

Importantly, the reported motives correspond to what we know about the use of stimulant drugs and similar substances today. We thus find consistency in how they have been used at least since the 1960s, possibly even longer (see Rasmussen, 2008). When addressing the distinction between medical and nonmedical use below, we will actually see some data allowing us to draw an even stronger conclusion. However, let us first relate what we have learned so far to the common illustration of the phenomenon in the media.

Neuroenhancement in the Media

It may be unlikely that, at least on a global level, a substantial number of students and other potential substance users actually follow scholarly debates in neuroethics. However, there is at least some agreement in the academic literature that the way enhancement is portrayed in the media affects people's expectations and decisions (see Coveney & Bjønness, 2019; Coveney et al., 2019; Partridge et al., 2011; Vargo & Petróczi, 2016). It has previously been argued that past hype, for example, about the possibilities of brain surgery and stimulation or psychopharmacological drugs, were fueled by optimistic accounts in popular media and that their portrayal of therapeutic options influenced patients' decisions (Racine et al., 2010; Schleim, 2014b; Snyder, 2009). The media thus seem to play an important role when it comes to informing potential consumers correctly and supporting "responsible use" (Greely et al., 2008).

However, the summary of past and recent prevalence surveys above has already put a big question mark behind the frequent portrayal of neuroenhancement as common and increasing. It goes without saying that there is also no fixed standard for when something is "common". In the debate among experts discussed above, Nora D. Volkow, director of the US National Institute on Drug Abuse, mentioned that 8% of 12th graders in the US had used amphetamine nonmedically in the previous year (Hyman et al., 2013). This number is accurate, and we will address it in a broader social and historical context in the next section. But does this figure, which might in many cases simply mean trying it out once, make nonmedical stimulant use *common?* We will look now in more detail at a few telling examples of how such figures are interpreted and presented.

For example, one study was repeatedly cited at the beginning of the enhancement debate, according to which 16% of students engaged in the practice (Babcock & Byrne, 2000). In addition to the poor methodological quality of this nonrepresentative survey, it also explicitly did *not* ask about cognitive performance enhancement but instead about the use of various drugs/medications "for fun". Another misleading interpretation referred to what was in itself a sound nationwide study conducted at various colleges in the US with a large number of participants (n = 10,904; McCabe et al., 2005), but focused on only *one* among the 119 educational institutions at which students were surveyed. At this single institution, 25% of respondents had answered "yes" to the question of whether they had used nonmedical prescription stimulants at least once in the past year, while, by comparison, this figure was 0% at 21 colleges and the average for all respondents across the 119 institutions was 4.1% (incidentally, this figure was only 2.1% for use in the past month).

Despite these findings, influential media outlets and even leading researchers repeatedly reported the 25% as if this applied to all (American) students. This is a very biased presentation of the scientific evidence, as it emphasizes extreme outliers that might simply reflect measurement problems and neglects important information about the frequency of substance use. Imagine throwing 119 darts at a board when blindfolded and then telling your friends only about the one single time you hit the "bull's eye". Moreover, this does not even take into account the fact that the study did not explicitly examine cognitive or neuroenhancement, but rather the broader concept of "non-medical use", as is common in such surveys (McCabe et al., 2005). Where the frequently reported figures of 16% and 25% of alleged nonmedical users come from is just one striking example of how the phenomenon has been and still is being turned misleadingly into an urgent problem.

There is no doubt that the media have a vested interest in generating a lot of attention. I analyze two examples from my own university's independent newspaper in Box 3.2 in detail to illustrate how the media construct such stories—and how they respond to critical remarks. My own past experience of following and writing about the topic for more than 15 years, as well as the limited scientific evidence available, indicate that such cases are not untypical (Partridge et al., 2011). However, even within academia, researchers are in competition with each other for research funding. Those who can convince their intended audience that they are tackling an urgent and societally relevant problem have an advantage over their competitors. In addition to questions of accuracy and honesty, adopting such a strategic approach could eventually lead to a situation where the public no longer believes science when it comes to real matters of life and death (such as climate change or infectious diseases).

Box 3.2 Examples from the Universiteitskrant of Groningen

The independent newspaper of the University of Groningen in the Netherlands has covered the topic of performance-enhancing substance use repeatedly over recent years, just like many other media outlets. The first of two examples I want to analyze here was presented as a "success story" in 2016 and described the collaboration between a medical and a business student.[6] The title already promised "better focus with a little pill". The text introduced the product as a "study pill" and linked it to the methylphenidate that students were allegedly increasingly using during exam periods. One of the founders of the company called "Braincaps" compared the product to Ritalin, but without the downsides. The article stated that due to the "overwhelming success", the entrepreneurs wanted to market their pills at places other than in Amsterdam and Groningen. One of their marketing methods was to put flyers on tables in the university library.

(continued)

---

[6] "Better focus with a little pill", *Universiteitskrant*, April 20, 2016, online at: https://archief.ukrant.nl/english/better-focus-with-a-little-pill-2.html

Box 3.2   (continued)

"Braincaps" still exists today.[7] The company is now based in a residential area in the small city of Apeldoorn. Neither the university newspaper then nor the company's website now refer to scientific studies about the product's effects. The website explains that it was tested by the company's owner and his former fellow students in Amsterdam. The primary product, "Braincaps Boost", is described as containing caffeine and theanine, thus substances also naturally found in coffee or green tea, as well as golden root (*Rhodiola rosea*). In the US, the *Food and Drug Administration* has warned several companies that have made false claims about the that plant's safety and efficacy.[8] For "Boost", theanine is described as increasing mental energy, but for their alternative product "Zen", it is described as relaxing. The products sell for €21.95 and €21.45, respectively, for 30 capsules. People could brew a lot coffee and tea at home for that amount of money.

At the time, I contacted the editors of the newspaper to argue that the evidence claims made in the article were implausible given the scientific literature (some of which we discussed earlier in this chapter). I pointed out that it was published right before the resits, and thus when students might be particularly desperate and vulnerable, leading them to try out new things, and I asked them to publish a comment based on my own research. The editor-in-chief turned down my request, explaining that the article was part of a series that was not focused on *what* students were selling, but *how* they were doing so. It was not the science, but the creative story behind it that mattered.[9]

The second example is more recent. In March 2021, the university newspaper published a feature article with the title, "Stimulant

(*continued*)

[7] https://www.braincaps.com/

[8] See https://www.fda.gov/inspections-compliance-enforcement-and-criminal--investigations/warning-letters/peak-nootropics-llc-aka-advanced-nootropics-557887-02052019

[9] Personal correspondence, April 25, 2016.

Box 3.2 (continued)

use is alarmingly high: What student doesn't love Ritalin?"[10] It referred to a survey carried out at my faculty by some of my colleagues (Fuermaier et al., 2021), allegedly showing "that a staggering 16 percent had taken methylphenidate". However, in the nonrepresentative sample of 1071 students, only *two* had stated that they did so regularly for nonmedical purposes, thus only 0.2%. Furthermore, the most frequent motive given was "leisure" and not in an "academic context". The 16% thus referred to lifetime prevalence and mostly reflected recreational use.

What happened next is—at the present moment—partially based on speculation, but it is likely that this article drew the attention of the secretary of state at the Dutch Ministry of Health, who sent a formal letter to the Dutch Parliament with the request to take measures to fight the use of ADHD medication among students for whom it was not intended. In his letter, he repeated the mistaken conclusion that "16% of the 1,071 surveyed students of the University of Groningen are using the medical drug Ritalin without a doctor's prescription to study".[11] Remember that this is based on a double confusion because, first, only 0.2% of the students were regular users (9.2% said they did so occasionally, which was not defined clearly), and, second, only a minority used it for academic purposes. Nonetheless, the university newspaper then wrote a follow-up article titled "Students need to stop using Ritalin as a study pill", describing the political intervention.[12] The article started with the unfounded statement that "[s]tudents are increasingly using drugs like Ritalin and Dextroamphetamine in order to focus" and repeated that,

(continued)

[10] *Universiteitskrant*, March 15, 2021, online at: https://ukrant.nl/magazine/what-student-doesnt-love-ritalin/?lang=en
[11] Paul Blokhuis's letter to the Dutch Parliament (*Tweede Kamer*) of November 15, 2021, correspondence number 3278642-1019312-GMT; my translation.
[12] *Universiteitskrant*, November 24, 2021, online at: https://ukrant.nl/students-need-to-stop-using-ritalin-as-a-study-pill/?lang=en

Box 3.2   (continued)

according to the study, "no fewer than 16 percent of first-year students take methylphenidate".

Again, I contacted the editors. They called the secretary's letter a reliable source, although that might have been biased by their own earlier misrepresentation. After a lengthy debate that went on for about a month, they at least distinguished between the figures for regular, occasional, and lifetime use in the articles and published a short interview with me—but only in Dutch, while the original article was also published in English.[13] It should be clear that such a correction will receive little attention weeks to months after the original exaggerating articles were published. The misrepresentation of primarily recreational as academic use was not corrected. After repeated invitations to comment on these issues, the editor-in-chief eventually replied that he felt not inclined to comment on a six-year-old story and further referred to the politician's letter.[14]

Meanwhile, the Dutch government started an initiative to fight the unintended use of ADHD medication. Based on a new but representative report, the figures in the Netherlands were found to be actually much lower than communicated by the university newspaper, with the past-month prevalence of 2.4% (men) and 1.5% (women) among students.[15] This is consistent with other surveys and the reviews we summarized above. We might at least consider the whole story as having a positive outcome, as the new Dutch Minister of Health and the initiative now aim to raise awareness for stress, coping issues, and performance pressure, as well as the guidelines for prescribing stimulant drugs.[16]

---

[13] *Universiteitskrant*, December 14, 2021, online at: https://ukrant.nl/ritalin-tegengaan-als-studiepil-is-niet-nodig/

[14] Personal correspondence, September 14, 2022.

[15] *Instituut Verantwoord Medicijngebruik*, "Gezonde focus: terugdringen van oneigenlijk gebruik van ADHD-medicatie", online at: https://www.tweedekamer.nl/downloads/document?id=2022D28239

[16] Ernst Kuipers's letter to the Dutch Parliament (*Tweede Kamer*) of June 30, 2022, correspondence number 3379693-1030624-GMT.

Medical or Nonmedical Use

Above, we discussed the paradox that substance users use the drugs in spite of scientific evidence that they are of no use. The best explanation for this incongruence was that researchers focused on cognitive factors, while the consumers took the stimulant drugs for their emotional and motivational effects. Now, we seem, again, to face a paradox: On the one hand, scholarly publications on neuroenhancement, as well as the general media, often exaggerate the phenomenon, while, on the other hand, the prevalence studies—with all their complexities and shortcomings—do not actually find the nonmedical use of prescription stimulants to be very common. This is particularly so under the narrower definition of academic performance enhancement.

As before, this prompts us to look differently at the data. Here, what we have learned in Chap. 2 about mental health and disorders, in combination with our theoretical considerations on how to distinguish disease, health, and enhancement, becomes useful. As a matter of fact, the production of the prescription stimulants of amphetamine and methylphenidate *has* increased greatly, particularly in the US (Fig. 3.2). Although the

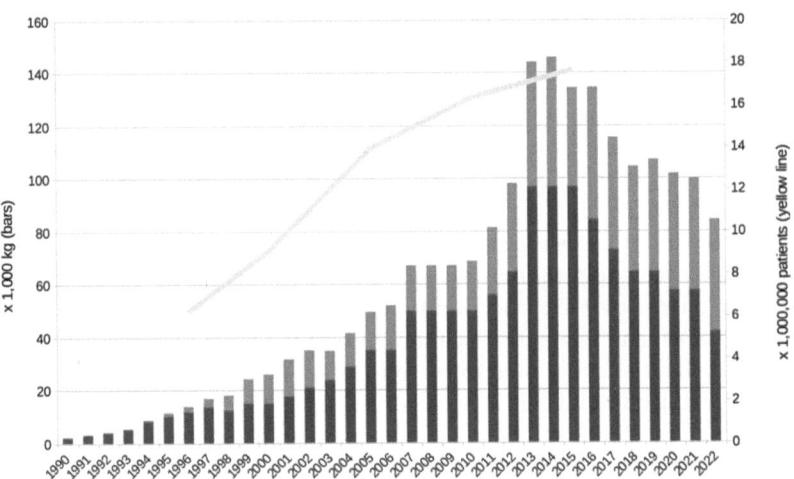

Fig. 3.2 Annual Production of Prescription Stimulants in the US. Since the 1990s, the annual production quotas of amphetamine (red) and methylphenidate (blue), as determined by the US government, increased greatly and reached a peak in 2014 (in 1000 kg, left scale). For comparison, the number of patients receiving antidepressants (yellow) in the US is shown here as well (in 1,000,000 patients, right scale). (Sources: *U.S. Federal Register*, Luo et al., 2020)

amounts have decreased somewhat after a peak in 2014, we were still seeing an *annual* production higher than that in the whole *decade* of the 1990s.

So, how can we reconcile the greatly increased production of stimulant drugs with the results of the surveys investigating the prevalence of their use? The answer has to do with what, by definition, the neuroenhancement debate and the surveys commonly are about: nonmedical use! This limited focus and framing ignored changes in the prevalence of ADHD diagnoses in children and adolescents, which in the US rose from about 6% in the late 1990s to 10% in the mid-2010s (Xu et al., 2018). These diagnoses often lead to the medical prescription of drugs containing amphetamine or methylphenidate (see also Bachmann et al., 2017) and are thus the best explanation for the increase in production.

There are also interesting cultural differences, with these prescription practices common in the Netherlands and the US but not in the UK, while Denmark and Germany lie somewhere in between (ibid.). This could be discussed along the rational of Chap. 2, that is, what kind of behavior is perceived as a medical problem (see also Singh & Wessely, 2015). The same goes for the fact that in the US, children with a white, non-Hispanic cultural background are much more likely to be given the diagnosis than others; and while children from poorer families are generally diagnosed more frequently, those from upper income families are most likely to receive prescription treatment (Xu et al., 2018). What is much more relevant in the present context is that after a long controversy, ADHD was eventually also acknowledged as a mental disorder common in adults and not only children and adolescents (Lange et al., 2010). This greatly increased the share of the population that could potentially receive the diagnosis and thus also the drugs.

It is difficult to fathom in detail what these changes in mental health care practices mean in a big country like the US, with more than 300 million citizens, and in a period spanning more than three decades. But it is obvious that the drugs prescribed to millions of people for daily use have to be produced—and this is what we see on Fig. 3.2. Researchers calculated that, for 2008, the supply of prescription stimulants for ADHD was sufficient to treat about 6.4 million individuals for all 365 days of the year (Swanson et al., 2011). Combining this with the official production quotas, we can estimate a theoretical upper boundary of 14 million *daily* users in the US in 2014! If they take the drugs on a doctor's prescription, none of them would appear in the prevalence studies discussed above, which explicitly exclude medical use.

Swanson and colleagues also pointed out that, in addition to the formation of large parental advocacy groups leading to the increasing recognition of the disorder since the late 1980s, the Individuals with Disabilities Education Act of 1990 included ADHD as an educational disability and made provisions for school-based services (ibid.). They argued that this explains at least part of the increase in diagnoses and prescriptions. In other words, getting the diagnosis became beneficial in certain school and academic settings. Even today, my own university gives students with an ADHD diagnosis 25% more time to complete an exam. Others have suggested that changes to the DSM criteria have also contributed to the increase (see, for example, Frances, 2013; Thomas et al., 2015).

However, for the present chapter, two other ideas are much more relevant: First of all, some people are feigning ADHD symptoms to receive the diagnosis and what they perceive as its associated benefits. This has actually prompted clinical psychologists at my own institute to develop methods to distinguish the "feigned" from the "real" disorder (Fuermaier et al., 2021; Tucha et al., 2015). Secondly, other people might knowingly or unknowingly eschew psychiatric diagnoses and use prescription or illicit drugs to treat their symptoms. This is discussed as "self-medication" in the literature (see, for example, Coveney et al., 2019; Lopes et al., 2015; Lucke et al., 2013).

Thus, reminiscent of the results of the previous chapters, the situation can be described as such: People using stimulants and saying "no" in the prevalence surveys (investigating nonmedical use) would have to answer "yes", *if* they feigned the symptoms successfully—or were misdiagnosed by a clinical expert. By contrast, people using stimulants and saying "yes" would have to answer "no", *if* their stimulant use is a valid case of self-medication. Recently, there has been increasing criticism of clinicians for diagnosing mental disorders too frequently and that general practitioners and psychiatrists prescribe too many psychopharmacological drugs (see Hengartner, 2022; Taylor, 2017). From this perspective, at least some "medical use" is mislabeled.

This apparently unlimited complexity has much to do with the theoretical as well as practical difficulty of distinguishing diseases/disorders, health/normalcy, and treatment/enhancement. The implication for the present question is that the available evidence cannot give a conclusive answer to whether nonmedical use of prescription stimulants—and other substances we will address in the next chapter—is increasing or decreasing. Above, we have at least discussed evidence from the 1960s to the 1980s which strongly suggests that nonmedical use—and with it neuroenhancement—has *not* become more common today. Given all these limitations, the best and realistically possible evidence would have to come from a longitudinal study asking people in the same situation, say, 12th graders, the same questions about their substance use over and over again. This is actually what the "Monitoring the Future" study at the University of Michigan has been doing for decades, again with the findings neglected by neuroethicists. Their results on amphetamine use without a doctor's prescription are shown on Fig. 3.3.

Above, we addressed the expert debate in which Nora Volkow referred to the 8% of 12th graders in the US that had been using amphetamine nonmedically in the previous year (Hyman et al., 2013). That was the situation in 2012, as we can see on the graph (Fig. 3.3). The much-lower 30-day prevalence of 3.3% in the same year confirms what we discussed

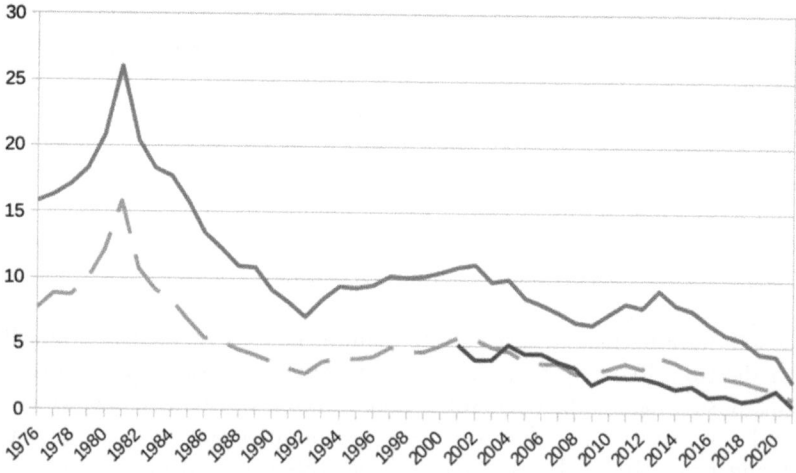

Fig. 3.3 Nonmedical Amphetamine Use of US 12th Graders. The graph shows the 12-month (red line) and 30-day prevalence (dashed orange line) of nonmedical amphetamine use among 12th graders in the US. The blue line shows the 12-month prevalence of nonmedical Ritalin use in the same group, which has been investigated for a shorter period of time. (Source: Monitoring the Future (Miech et al., 2022))

above: Most of these students are not regular users. However, the graph actually illustrates three more important findings: Firstly, also in line with our previous discussion, nonmedical use is less frequent than in the 1970s and 1980s. Secondly, although there was a slight rebound effect from the preliminary low in 1992 until 2002, the overall negative trend persists until today. Thirdly, the further substantial decrease from 4.3% in 2020 to 2.3% in 2021 suggests the common recreational use of the drug: During pandemic-related lockdowns and periods of home schooling, the emotional/motivational demands on students remained high, but they had fewer opportunities to go out and have fun with their peers.

We can thus conclude with considerable certainty that the nonmedical consumption of stimulant drugs has been decreasing continuously and that much of that use is recreational. This clearly contradicts the frequently communicated message that neuroenhancement is common and increasing (see also Partridge et al., 2011; Schleim & Quednow, 2018). It further shows how misleading headlines and descriptions in the media are when they suggest that almost all students are taking drugs to improve their academic performance (Box 3.2). As we saw above, on the basis of misrepresented data, the Dutch government recently launched an initiative to fight the nonintended use of ADHD medication in the country. But is there really much to fight, if the last-month prevalence is as low as what is shown in the last figure?

3.3   Nonpharmacological Alternatives

Substance use is obviously the focus of this book. However, when one discusses a phenomenon, knowing more about its alternatives often improves one's understanding as well. With respect to the broader topic of mental health and enhancement, learning more about nonpharmacological options is also informative and helpful. We have already seen above that researchers summarizing the neuroenhancement debate have pointed to "biobehavioral strategies" as complementary ways to enhance cognition (Dresler et al., 2019; see also Dresler et al., 2013). They listed physical exercise, sleep, meditation, learning a new language, mnemonics (i.e., specific techniques to improve one's memory), and computer training as such strategies.

Other researchers have described the beneficial effects of physical exercise on the brain as well (Hötting & Röder, 2013). They emphasized our greater understanding of how the nervous system is affected by physical training, particularly regarding an increase in neuroplasticity. This refers to the brain's capacity to respond to the demands of people's life situations, resulting in long-lasting structural changes. The benefits, Hötting and Röder explain, could be maximized through a combination of cognitive training and overall cardiovascular fitness.

Linking the book's general topic with this section on alternatives in a convenient way, Caviola and Faber compared computer-assisted learning, sleep, and exercise more specifically with pharmacological neuroenhancement (Caviola & Faber, 2015). We have already seen in the discussion above that the experimental evidence in favor of that is ambiguous. This, of course, in itself limits comparability with alternative approaches. However, according to this specific review, people who do not take the drugs at least do not seem to miss out on beneficial effects:

> We find that all of the techniques described can produce significant beneficial effects on cognitive performance. However, effect sizes are moderate, and consistently dependent on individual and situational factors as well as the cognitive domain in question. [...] [W]e can conclude that pharmacological cognitive enhancement is not more effective than non-pharmacological cognitive enhancement. (Caviola & Faber, 2015, p. 1)

Psychology in general has, of course, a long history of understanding memory, learning, and intelligence. While this body of research is much too vast to be summarized here, Roger N. Walsh, professor of psychiatry, philosophy, and anthropology at the University of California, Irvine, has reviewed knowledge about the relation between lifestyle and mental health that has proved useful as a complement to psychotherapy (Walsh, 2011). He, along with many other researchers, also describes the benefits of physical exercise for multiple body systems and even cognitive improvement. Walsh particularly points to physical exercise as a means to both prevent and treat mild to moderate depression. Nutrition and diet are important factors as well, comprising food selection and supplements. Spending time in nature is also being increasingly investigated for its beneficial effects and contrasted with unbalanced media immersion, such as spending too much time watching television or using digital media.

There are many more factors that are actually reminiscent of the "pillars of health" that we discussed briefly in the introduction. Walsh also reviews the important role of relationships, recreation and enjoyable activities, relaxation and stress management, religious and spiritual involvement, as well as contribution and service (Walsh, 2011). He thus advocates a very comprehensive account of health and well-being. By contrast, a strong emphasis on more physiological aspects such as healthy diet, sufficient physical exercise, and avoiding unhealthy substance use has generally drawn attention away from the importance of social relationships and integration, in spite of their strong effects on mortality (Holt-Lunstad et al., 2010). Social psychologists have confirmed that many people underestimate the importance of social factors (Haslam et al., 2018).

Neurotechnology in general or substance use in particular may seem so attractive to many because these strategies "do the work for us", so to speak. Most, if not all, of the abovementioned alternatives demand our time and attention. The more commonly discussed ways to achieve neuroenhancement can simply be applied (e.g., brain stimulation) or consumed (e.g., substances), even if they still come at a financial cost. Perhaps it helps us here to realize that our present bodies are the product of a long evolutionary history with their selection and survival pressures, which can be understood as a continuous process of adaptation and optimization. This implies that if there were simple ways to make us even more efficient, they probably would have evolved naturally. That the neuroenhancement debate has, after 20 years, been unable to identify a real "game changer" might simply testify to the fact that we are already functioning on a very high level, perhaps even at too high a level, considering the negative consequences of human action on the global scale. These thoughts remind us that the time is ripe for a general conclusion to this chapter.

3.4   INTERIM CONCLUSION: HYPE OR REALITY?

At the beginning of this chapter, we situated the neuroenhancement debate in the competitive performance society of the early twenty-first century. Our time's obsession with measuring, comparing, ranking, and then optimizing everything is characteristic of it. In the sections that followed, we discussed data and findings that make more sense in this context than that suggested by neuroethicists. I am actually aware of no evidence at all indicating that a considerable number of students are taking drugs based on their own will to become smarter, to become a "little Einstein". This also makes sense in light of the tentative conclusion that— at least in healthy consumers without sleep deprivation—stimulant drugs primarily affect emotion and motivation, not cognition.

Ethicists have repeatedly emphasized the importance of considering both safety and coercion. However, regarding the former, it has to be conceded that even after some 20 years of research and debate there is still no reliable data on the consequences of the long-term use of these drugs. Moreover, neuroethicists cannot complain that there has been a lack of funding for their endeavor. By contrast, it was a booming field with numerous research projects and opportunities around the globe. The conclusion is less obvious with respect to coercion, also because it is complex to decide at what point tolerable pressure becomes intolerable coercion. Yet, we do have some reliable and consistent qualitative, as well as quantitative, evidence that competition and performance pressure increase students' likelihood of taking prescription stimulants—whether we label this medical or nonmedical use. Their practice primarily seems to be a way of increasing their motivation and coping with stress. While some individuals might prefer to reflect on whether they are in the right environment, we should also critically analyze what that environment is like, what it demands of people, and which behaviors it rewards or punishes.

The recent reviews by Dresler et al. (2019) and Racine et al. (2021) are helpful in that they summarize and systematize a large part of the debate on neuroenhancement and make useful suggestions for future research. However, their accounts also emphasize the sheer complexity of this approach by identifying numerous factors that have been insufficiently addressed over the past 20 years. It is presently unclear whether another 20 years would yield a substantially different outcome other than concluding (again) that the questions are more complex than previously thought.

Here, we should also mention the possibility of a serious conflict of interest: In neuroethics, so to speak, a distinct group of people identifies the topics that are relevant and thus define the agenda on ethical, legal, and social issues related to neuroscience. Many major research initiatives on the brain currently have dedicated funds for research of this kind (Amadio et al., 2018). The people setting the research agenda in advance are thus the same as those eventually employed to carry out the investigations. But what might the agenda look like if it was determined in a democratic decision-making process? Would people value neuroenhancement higher than, say, good housing, fair employment, and a safe environment? The strong emphasis on cognitive performance might simply misrepresent the priorities of the majority of people (Schleim, 2014a) and doesn't even seem to match the priorities of these professors' own students (see Vargo & Petróczi, 2016; Vrecko, 2013).

Raymond De Vries and Fernando Vidal were two of the very few investigating these structural issues concerning the preconditions of a field such as neuroethics (De Vries, 2007; Vidal, 2018). We thus face a reiteration of the "Who watches the watchdog?" problem. That this not only matters theoretically can be illustrated by the fact that, in contrast to the common narrative in neuroethics, enhancement is emotional rather cognitive, moral enhancement is not new, and nonmedical stimulant use is decreasing not increasing. This book is not meant as an exercise in the sociology of science, as important a field as that may be. But understanding the structure of an area of research helps us to understand the answers it can provide and the knowledge that it creates.

Instead of pursuing these questions here any further, we will stick to our topic. With respect to neuroethics—or at least neuroenhancement—the conclusion seems that *the hype is the reality*. That is, old trends of substance use have been reframed using different words—enhancement—and then put on the research agenda with the help of powerful media partners. Whether and when the "neuroenhancement bubble" (Lucke et al., 2011; see also ter Meulen et al., 2017) bursts, depends on the decisions of researchers and their funders. Considering this conclusion in combination with the persistent inability to draw clear lines between disorder/disease, health/normalcy, and enhancement, it seems justified for us to look at substances independent of mental disorder categories and to drop the concepts of cognitive and neuroenhancement altogether. This thus paves the way for a fresh look at substance use in the next chapter.

REFERENCES

Agay, N., Yechiam, E., Carmel, Z., & Levkovitz, Y. (2010). Non-specific effects of methylphenidate (Ritalin) on cognitive ability and decision-making of ADHD and healthy adults. *Psychopharmacology, 210,* 511–519.

Amadio, J., Bi, G.-Q., Boshears, P. F., Carter, A., Devor, A., Doya, K., et al. (2018). Neuroethics questions to guide ethical research in the international brain initiatives. *Neuron, 100,* 19–36.

Babcock, Q., & Byrne, T. (2000). Student perceptions of methylphenidate abuse at a public liberal arts college. *Journal of American College Health, 49,* 143–145.

Bachmann, C. J., Wijlaars, L. P., Kalverdijk, L. J., Burcu, M., Glaeske, G., Schuiling-Veninga, C. C. M., Hoffmann, F., Aagaard, L., & Zito, J. M. (2017). Trends in ADHD medication use in children and adolescents in five western countries, 2005–2012. *European Neuropsychopharmacology, 27,* 484–493.

Battleday, R. M., & Brem, A. K. (2015). Modafinil for cognitive neuroenhancement in healthy non-sleep-deprived subjects: A systematic review. *European Neuropsychopharmacology, 25*, 1865–1881.

Beddington, J., Cooper, C. L., Field, J., Goswami, U., Huppert, F. A., Jenkins, R., Jones, H. S., Kirkwood, T. B. L., Sahakian, B. J., & Thomas, S. M. (2008). The mental wealth of nations. *Nature, 455*, 1057–1060.

Caviola, L., & Faber, N. S. (2015). Pills or push-ups? effectiveness and public perception of pharmacological and non-pharmacological cognitive enhancement. *Frontiers in Psychology, 6*, 1852.

Compton, W. M., Han, B., Blanco, C., Johnson, K., & Jones, C. M. (2018). Preva-lence and correlates of prescription stimulant use, misuse, use disorders, and motivations for misuse among adults in the United States. *American Journal of Psychiatry, 175*, 741–755.

Coveney, C., & Bjønness, J. (2019). Making sense of pharmaceutical cognitive enhancement: Taking stock and looking forward. *Drugs: Education, Prevention and Policy, 26*, 293–300.

Coveney, C., Williams, S. J., & Gabe, J. (2019). Enhancement imaginaries: Exploring public understandings of pharmaceutical cognitive enhancing drugs. *Drugs: Education. Prevention and Policy, 26*, 319–328.

De Vries, R. (2007). Who will guard the guardians of neuroscience? *EMBO Reports, 8*, S65–S69.

Delgado, J. M. R. (1971). *Physical control of the mind: Toward a psychocivilized society.* Harper & Row.

Delgado, J. M. R. (1983). The psychophysiology of freedom. *Political Psychology, 4*, 355–374.

DeSantis, A., Noar, S. M., & Webb, E. M. (2009). Nonmedical ADHD stimulant use in fraternities. *Journal of Studies on Alcohol and Drugs, 70*, 952–954.

Douglas, T. (2008). Moral Enhancement. *Journal of Applied Philosophy, 25*(3), 228–245.

Dresler, M., Sandberg, A., Bublitz, C., Ohla, K., Trenado, C., Mroczko-Wąsowicz, A., Kühn, S., & Repantis, D. (2019). Hacking the brain: Dimensions of cognitive enhancement. *ACS Chemical Neuroscience, 10*, 1137–1148.

Dresler, M., Sandberg, A., Ohla, K., Bublitz, C., Trenado, C., Mroczko-Wąsowicz, A., Kühn, S., & Repantis, D. (2013). Non-pharmacological cognitive enhancement. *Neuropharmacology, 64*, 529–543.

Elliott, G. R., & Elliott, M. D. (2011). Pharmacological cognitive enhancers: Comment on Smith and Farah (2011). *Psychological Bulletin, 137*, 749–750.

Farah, M. J. (2015). The unknowns of cognitive enhancement. *Science, 350*, 379–380.

Farah, M. J., Illes, J., Cook-Deegan, R., Gardner, H., Kandel, E., King, P., Parens, E., Sahakian, B., & Wolpe, P. R. (2004). Neurocognitive enhancement: What can we do and what should we do? *Nature Reviews Neuroscience, 5*, 421–425.

Faraone, S. V., Rostain, A. L., Montano, C. B., Mason, O., Antshel, K. M., & Newcorn, J. H. (2020). Systematic review: Nonmedical use of prescription stimulants: Risk factors, outcomes, and risk reduction strategies. *Journal of the American Academy of Child and Adolescent Psychiatry, 59*, 100–112.

Fins, J. J., & Vernaglia, J. S. (2022). Jose Manuel Rodriguez Delgado, Walter Freeman, and psychosurgery: A study in contrasts. *Neuroscientist.* https://doi.org/10.1177/10738584221086603

Frances, A. (2013). *Saving normal: An insider's revolt against out-of-control psychiatric diagnosis, DSM-5, Big Pharma, and the medicalization of ordinary life.* William Morrow.

Franke, A. G., Gransmark, P., Agricola, A., Schuhle, K., Rommel, T., Sebastian, A., Balló, H. E., Gorbulev, S., Gerdes, C., Frank, B., Ruckes, C., Tüscher, O., & Lieb, K. (2017). Methylphenidate, modafinil, and caffeine for cognitive enhancement in chess: A double-blind, randomised controlled trial. *European Neuropsychopharmacology, 27*, 248–260.

Fuermaier, A. B. M., Tucha, O., Koerts, J., Tucha, L., Thome, J., & Faltraco, F. (2021). Feigning ADHD and stimulant misuse among Dutch university students. *Journal of Neural Transmission, 128*, 1079–1084.

Greely, H., Sahakian, B., Harris, J., Kessler, R. C., Gazzaniga, M., Campbell, P., & Farah, M. J. (2008). Towards responsible use of cognitive-enhancing drugs by the healthy. *Nature, 456*, 702–705.

Greene, J. D., Nystrom, L. E., Engell, A. D., Darley, J. M., & Cohen, J. D. (2004). The neural bases of cognitive conflict and control in moral judgment. *Neuron, 44*, 389–400.

Haslam, S. A., McMahon, C., Cruwys, T., Haslam, C., Jetten, J., & Steffens, N. K. (2018). Social cure, what social cure? The propensity to underestimate the importance of social factors for health. *Social Science & Medicine, 198*, 14–21.

Heinz, A., & Müller, S. (2017). Exaggerating the benefits and downplaying the risks in the bioethical debate on cognitive neuroenhancement. In R. ter Meulen, A. D. Mohamed, & W. Hall (Eds.), *Rethinking cognitive enhancement* (pp. 69–86). Oxford University Press.

Hengartner, M. P. (2022). *Evidence-biased antidepressant prescription: Overmedicalisation, flawed research, and conflicts of interest.* Palgrave Macmillan.

Holt-Lunstad, J., Smith, T. B., & Layton, J. B. (2010). Social relationships and mortality risk: A meta-analytic review. *PLoS Medicine, 7*(7), e1000316.

Hope, V. D., Underwood, M., Mulrooney, K., Mazanov, J., van de Ven, K., & McVeigh, J. (2021). Human enhancement drugs: Emerging issues and responses. *International Journal of Drug Policy, 95*, 103459.

Hötting, K., & Röder, B. (2013). Beneficial effects of physical exercise on neuroplasticity and cognition. *Neuroscience & Biobehavioral Reviews, 37*, 2243–2257.

Hyman, S., Volkow, N., & Nutt, D. (2013). Pharmacological cognitive enhancement in healthy people: Potential and concerns. *Neuropharmacology, 64,* 8–12.

Ilieva, I. P., & Farah, M. J. (2013). Enhancement stimulants: Perceived motivational and cognitive advantages. *Frontiers in Neuroscience, 7,* 198.

Ilieva, I. P., & Farah, M. J. (2019). Attention, Motivation, and Study Habits in Users of Unprescribed ADHD Medication. *Journal of Attention Disorders, 23,* 149–162.

Inon, M. (2019). Fooled by 'smart drugs'—why shouldn't pharmacological cognitive enhancement be liberally used in education? *Ethics and Education, 14,* 54–69.

Juengst, E., & Moseley, D. (2019). Human enhancement. In: Edward N. Zalta (ed.), *The Stanford Encyclopedia of Philosophy* (Summer 2019 Edition). URL = https://plato.stanford.edu/archives/sum2019/entries/enhancement/

Kaufman, K. R. (2005). Modafinil in sports: Ethical considerations. *British Journal of Sports Medicine, 39,* 241–244.

Lange, K. W., Reichl, S., Lange, K. M., Tucha, L., & Tucha, O. (2010). The history of attention deficit hyperactivity disorder. *ADHD Attention Deficit and Hyperactivity Disorders, 2,* 241–255.

Langlitz, N., Dyck, E., Scheidegger, M., & Repantis, D. (2021). Moral psychopharmacology needs moral inquiry: The case of psychedelics. *Frontiers in Psychiatry, 12,* 680064.

Lopes, N., Clamote, T., Raposo, H., Pegado, E., & Rodrigues, C. (2015). Medications, youth therapeutic cultures and performance consumptions: A sociological approach. *Health, 19,* 430–448.

Lucke, J., Partridge, B., & Hall, W. (2013). Dealing with Ennui: To what extent is "cognitive enhancement" a form of self-medication for symptoms of depression? *AJOB Neuroscience, 4,* 17–17.

Lucke, J. C., Bell, S., Partridge, B., & Hall, W. D. (2011). Deflating the neuroenhancement bubble. *AJOB Neuroscience, 2,* 38–43.

Luo, Y., Kataoka, Y., Ostinelli, E. G., Cipriani, A., & Furukawa, T. A. (2020). National prescription patterns of antidepressants in the treatment of adults with major depression in the US between 1996 and 2015: A population representative survey based analysis. *Frontiers in Psychiatry, 11,* 35.

Maier, L. J., Ferris, J. A., & Winstock, A. R. (2018). Pharmacological cognitive enhancement among non-ADHD individuals-A cross-sectional study in 15 countries. *International Journal of Drug Policy, 58,* 104–112.

McAuliffe, W. E., Rohman, M., Fishman, P., Friedman, R., Wechsler, H., Soboroff, S. H., & Toth, D. (1984). Psychoactive drug-use by young and future physicians. *Journal of Health and Social Behavior, 25,* 34–54.

McAuliffe, W. E., Rohman, M., Santangelo, S., Feldman, B., Magnuson, E., Sobol, A., & Weissman, J. (1986). Psychoactive drug use among practicing physicians and medical students. *New England Journal of Medicine,* *315,* 805–810.

McCabe, S. E., Teter, C. J., Boyd, C. J., Knight, J. R., & Wechsler, H. (2005). Nonmedical use of prescription opioids among U.S. college students: Prevalence and correlates from a national survey. *Addictive Behaviors, 30,* 789–805.

McCabe, S. E., West, B. T., Teter, C. J., & Boyd, C. J. (2014). Trends in medical use, diversion, and nonmedical use of prescription medications among college students from 2003 to 2013: Connecting the dots. *Addictive Behaviors, 39,* 1176–1182.

Miech, R. A., Johnston, L. D., O'Malley, P. M., Bachman, J. G., Schulenberg, J. E., & Patrick, M. E. (2022). *Monitoring the future national survey results on drug use, 1975–2021: Volume I, Secondary school students.* Institute for Social Research, The University of Michigan.

Müller, U., Rowe, J. B., Rittman, T., Lewis, C., Robbins, T. W., & Sahakian, B. J. (2013). Effects of modafinil on non-verbal cognition, task enjoyment and creative thinking in healthy volunteers. *Neuropharmacology, 64,* 490–495.

O'Connor, C., Rees, G., & Joffe, H. (2012). Neuroscience in the Public Sphere. *Neuron, 74,* 220–226.

Partridge, B. J., Bell, S. K., Lucke, J. C., Yeates, S., & Hall, W. D. (2011). Smart drugs "as common as coffee": Media hype about neuroenhancement. *PLOS ONE, 6,* e28416.

President's Council on Bioethics. (2003). *Beyond therapy: Biotechnology and the pursuit of happiness.* Dana Press.

Quednow, B. B. (2010). Ethics of neuroenhancement: A phantom debate. *BioSocieties, 5,* 153–156.

Racine, E., Sattler, S., & Boehlen, W. (2021). Cognitive enhancement: Unanswered questions about human psychology and social behavior. *Science and Engineering Ethics, 27,* 19.

Racine, E., Waldman, S., Rosenberg, J., & Illes, J. (2010). Contemporary neuroscience in the media. *Social Science & Medicine, 71,* 725–733.

Rasmussen, N. (2008). *On Speed: The many lives of amphetamine.* New York University Press.

Schleim, S. (2010). Second thoughts on the prevalence of enhancement. *BioSocieties, 5*(4), 484–485.

Schleim, S. (2011). Glück in der Psychopharmakologie: Affektives und kognitives Enhancement. In D. Thomä, C. Henning & O. Mitscherlich (Eds.), *Glück: Ein interdisziplinäres Handbuch* (pp. 383–387). Stuttgart: Metzler.

Schleim, S. (2014a). Whose well-being? Common conceptions and misconceptions in the enhancement debate. *Frontiers in Systems Neuroscience, 8,* 148.

Schleim, S. (2014b). Critical neuroscience—or critical science? a perspective on the perceived normative significance of neuroscience. *Frontiers in Human Neuroscience, 8,* 336.

Schleim, S. (2020a). Real neurolaw in the Netherlands: The role of the developing brain in the new adolescent criminal law. *Frontiers in Psychology, 11*, 1762.

Schleim, S. (2020b). Neuroenhancement as instrumental drug use: Putting the debate in a different frame. *Frontiers in Psychiatry, 11*, 567497.

Schleim, S. (2021). Neurorights in history: A contemporary review of José M. R. Delgado's "Physical Control of the Mind" (1969) and Elliot S. Valenstein's "Brain Control" (1973). *Frontiers in Human Neuroscience, 15*, 615.

Schleim, S. (2022a). Grounded in biology: Why the context-dependency of psychedelic drug effects means opportunities, not problems for anthropology and pharmacology. *Frontiers in Psychiatry, 13*, 906487.

Schleim, S. (2022b). *Pharmacological enhancement: The facts and myths about brain doping.* Theory and History of Psychology, University of Groningen.

Schleim, S., & Quednow, B. B. (2017). Debunking the ethical neuroenhancement debate. In R. ter Meulen, A. D. Mohamed, & W. Hall (Eds.), *Rethinking cognitive enhancement: A critical appraisal of the neuroscience and ethics of cognitive enhancement* (pp. 164–175). Oxford University Press.

Schleim, S., & Quednow, B. B. (2018). How realistic are the scientific assumptions of the neuroenhancement debate? assessing the pharmacological optimism and neuroenhancement prevalence hypotheses. *Frontiers in Pharmacology, 9*, 3.

Singh, I., Bard, I., & Jackson, J. (2014). Robust resilience and substantial interest: A survey of pharmacological cognitive enhancement among university students in the UK and Ireland. *PLOS ONE, 9*, e105969.

Singh, I., & Wessely, S. (2015). Childhood: A suitable case for treatment? *The Lancet Psychiatry, 2*, 661–666.

Skinner, B. F. (1971). *Beyond freedom and dignity.* Hackett Publishing.

Smith, M. E., & Farah, M. J. (2011). Are prescription stimulants "smart pills"? The epidemiology and cognitive neuroscience of prescription stimulant use by normal healthy individuals. *Psychological Bulletin, 137*, 717–741.

Snyder, P. (2009). Delgado's brave bulls: The marketing of a seductive idea and a lesson for contemporary biomedical research. In P. Snyder, L. Mayes, & D. Spencer (Eds.), *Science and the media: Delgado's brave bull and the ethics of scientific disclosure* (pp. 25–40). Academic Press.

Somit, A. (Ed.). (1976). *Biology and politics: Recent explorations.* De Gruyter Mouton.

Swanson, J. M., Wigal, T. L., & Volkow, N. D. (2011). Contrast of medical and nonmedical use of stimulant drugs, basis for the distinction, and risk of addiction: Comment on Smith and Farah (2011). *Psychological Bulletin, 137*, 742–748.

Taylor, E. (2017). Attention deficit hyperactivity disorder: Overdiagnosed or diagnoses missed? *Archives of Disease in Childhood, 102*, 376–379.

ter Meulen, R. H. J., Mohamed, A. D., & Hall, W. (2017). *Rethinking cognitive enhancement*. Oxford University Press.

Teter, C. J., Falone, A. E., Cranford, J. A., Boyd, C. J., & McCabe, S. E. (2010). Nonmedical use of prescription stimulants and depressed mood among college students: Frequency and routes of administration. *Journal of Substance Abuse Treatment, 38*, 292–298.

Thomas, R., Sanders, S., Doust, J., Beller, E., & Glasziou, P. (2015). Prevalence of attention-deficit/hyperactivity disorder: A systematic review and meta-analysis. *Pediatrics, 135*, e994–e1001.

Tucha, L., Fuermaier, A. B. M., Koerts, J., Groen, Y., & Thome, J. (2015). Detection of feigned attention deficit hyperactivity disorder. *Journal of Neural Transmission, 122*, 123–134.

Turner, D., & Sahakian, B. (2006). The cognition-enhanced classroom. In P. Miller & J. Wilsdon (Eds.), *Better Humans? The politics of human enhancement and life extension* (pp. 79–85). Demos.

Valenstein, E. S. (1974). *Brain control*. Wiley.

Vargo, E. J., & Petróczi, A. (2016). "It was me on a good day": Exploring the smart drug use phenomenon in England. *Frontiers in Psychology, 7*, 779.

Vidal, F. (2018). What makes neuroethics possible? *History of the Human Sciences, 32*, 32–58.

Vidal, F., & Piperberg, M. (2017). Born free: The theory and practice of neuro-ethical exceptionalism. In E. Racine & J. Aspler (Eds.), *Debates about neuroethics: Perspectives on its development, focus, and future* (pp. 67–81). Springer International Publishing.

Vrecko, S. (2013). Just how cognitive is "Cognitive Enhancement"? On the significance of emotions in university students' experiences with study drugs. *AJOB Neuroscience, 4*, 4–12.

Walsh, R. (2011). Lifestyle and mental health. *American Psychologist, 66*, 579–592.

Wilfond, B. S., & Ravitsky, V. (2005). On the proliferation of bioethics sub-disciplines: Do we really need "genethics" and "neuroethics"? *The American Journal of Bioethics, 5*, 20–21.

Xu, G., Strathearn, L., Liu, B., Yang, B., & Bao, W. (2018). Twenty-Year trends in diagnosed attention-deficit/hyperactivity disorder among US children and adolescents, 1997–2016. *JAMA Network Open, 1*, e181471–e181471.

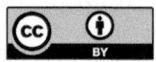

CHAPTER 4

Substance Use

The fundamental urge to alter our consciousness in significant but controllable ways is, it seems, part of our hard-wiring. Very few people live their lives without using some kind of mind-altering substance, be it a cup of coffee, a glass of wine, sleeping pills, cigarettes or betel.
—Ken Arnold, *Head of Public Programmes, Wellcome Collection, London (in: Jay, 2010, p. 6)*

Abstract This chapter starts out with a theoretical discussion of the meaning of "drug". As it turns out, three different kinds of psychoactive drugs can be distinguished. Central to this distinction is the understanding of appropriate medical use, which is subject to change. Historical examples illustrate how our personal and also governments' ways to think about drugs changed since the nineteenth century. In the past, colonial authorities were the biggest drug traders and countries even waged war to enforce open markets. Cocaine, opium, and nitrous oxide (laughing gas) are addressed in detail. The legal regulation of that last substance even changed as the book was being written. The framework for people's instrumental substance use is then introduced. It distinguishes different reasons for which drugs can be instrumentalized. Several common substances are described subsequently, addressing their respective risks and benefits. The final section presents important values that can guide moral decisions about drug use.

© The Author(s) 2023
S. Schleim, *Mental Health and Enhancement*, Palgrave Studies in
Law, Neuroscience, and Human Behavior,
https://doi.org/10.1007/978-3-031-32618-9_4

Keywords Drugs • Drug policy • Alcohol • Opium • Cocaine •
Nitrous oxide • Instrumental substance use • Drug instrumentalization

We have just concluded that there are no clear boundaries between disorder/disease, health/normality, and enhancement. This does not deny that there are many individual cases which we can meaningfully identify as either disease (e.g., a malignant tumor) or enhancement (e.g., implants to equip people with infrared vision). However, the inability to find clear definitions of these concepts becomes highly relevant in this chapter on substance use. After all, the legal distinction between licit and illicit drugs, between freely available substances and regulated drugs, depends very much on whether medical and administrative authorities consider them as a valid treatment for a medical disease or mental disorder. With what we have learned in Chap. 2, we can say that these decisions are examples of pragmatism and social constructionism, but that they are also guided by the drugs' intrinsic properties, which reflects essentialism (see also Schleim, 2018).

The classifications eventually made and maintained by the authorities responsible for drug policy can and do have serious consequences for many people: Will they have access to a substance legally, or do they risk being sentenced, in severe cases to years in prison, merely for its possession? By avoiding the reification of present distinctions between licit and illicit drugs, we can better understand how this system evolved in the twentieth century. The first section of this chapter will thus discuss the theoretical difference between nutritional supplements, natural stimulants (such as alcohol, coffee, and tobacco), licit, and illicit drugs. This is then exemplified with a couple of illustrative historical cases in the second section. The subsequent section on instrumental use will systematize the topic of this chapter, and to a certain extent the whole book, from the present perspective. The final section discusses different values that may underlie and guide decisions on substance use.

4.1   Kinds of Substances

Substances—think of the sugar extracted from sugarcane or beet, the caffeine in coffee beans, the cocaine extracted from coca leaves, or the methylphenidate synthesized from other chemical compounds—do not come with a label telling us what they are good (or bad) for. Their effects and side effects are something we humans have to find out for ourselves. The distinction between natural and unnatural means, which often plays a role in ethical debates, does not help us much. Just as natural substances can have therapeutic effects when used properly—such as St. John's wort (*Hypericum perforatum*), which has been found to be similarly effective in treating mild-to-moderate depression as some of the frequently prescribed pharmaceutical drugs used today (Ng et al., 2017)—there are also many poisons in nature. Furthermore, the wisdom of Paracelsus (c. 1493–1541), who said that "the dose makes the poison", is still valid and illustrates once more that a spectrum of distinctions is much more appropriate than concepts that suggest clear borders.

Similar to the analysis of the history and meaning of "addiction" in Chap. 2, we should spend some time in this chapter looking at where the present classification system of substances comes from and what this "present system" is after all. When preparing this section, I had the problem, for example, that there is no direct corresponding term in many languages for the German term *Genussmittel* or the Dutch *genotmiddel*, literally meaning something that is consumed for enjoyment or as a mild stimulant (see Hengartner & Merki, 1999; Schivelbusch, 2010). In debates on drug policy, this term often functions to positively frame substances not primarily consumed for their nutritional value, while distinguishing them from the "bad drugs" (*Droge* or *drug* in the two languages).

Some English dictionaries translate *Genussmittel* as "(natural) stimulant" (similar to the Spanish *el estimulante*, for example), while others just list a number of substances: "alcoholic drinks, coffee, tea, tobacco, etc." We call the latter an "enumerative definition" in philosophy, which is commonly used when we have no better idea about what to call something. People and cultures in different times would probably disagree on what to add to the list (see Goodman et al., 2007). Speaking of "stimulants", by contrast, has the downside of blurring the line with the strictly regulated stimulant drugs we discussed in detail in the previous chapter. Furthermore, this would not do justice to the fact that the consumption of alcohol beyond a certain threshold quickly leads to severe impairment of cognitive functioning.

Three Kinds of Drugs

That the English language knows no equivalent for *Genussmittel* may explain the ambiguity of its term "drug". Some link its etymology to Old

French *drogue* (Tupper, 2012), meaning "any substance, of animal, vegetable, or mineral origin, used as an ingredient in pharmacy, chemistry, dyeing, or various manufacturing processes" (ibid., p. 465). As an extension of this, the *Oxford Dictionary of English* (online edition) relates it to Dutch *droog*, literally meaning "dry", referring to dried, often colonial goods, sold in the "drug store" even today (Dutch *drogisterij*, German *Drogerie*). Kenneth W. Tupper, a researcher on psychedelic substances and adjunct professor of population and public health at the University of British Columbia in Canada, distinguishes three meanings of "drug" in contemporary English, referred to as $drug_1$, $drug_2$, and $drug_3$.

The first is synonymous with "medicine" and contains substances which are psychoactive or not. Tupper explains that when coca products and opium were increasingly marketed as "drugs" in the early twentieth century, pharmacists in the US launched a concerted campaign to preserve this term for medicine in the more narrow sense (Tupper, 2012; see also Parascandola, 1995). Roughly 100 years later, we now know that this failed. The meaning of $drug_2$ is "a chemical substance other than a food that alters consciousness when absorbed into the body" (Tupper, 2012, p. 466). The focus here thus lies on the psychoactive effects, also reflected in the phrase "to drug someone". Some of these substances can be medicines in the sense of $drug_1$, others can be legal but regulated, such as alcohol, and yet others can be prohibited, such as cocaine and heroin. The meaning of $drug_2$ is thus independent of the legal status of the substance.

This is different for $drug_3$, which refers to "a plant or chemical substance that alters human consciousness and has been subjected to the most rigorous forms of control—typically criminalization—under the international drug control regime" (ibid., p. 467). $Drugs_3$ are thus the *prohibited* subset of $drugs_2$, and this idea reflects how *Droge* or *drug* are commonly, perhaps even exclusively, used in German or Dutch, respectively. Almost all substances discussed in this book are drugs in the sense of $drug_2$, because of the way they interact with the human nervous system. An exception are those substances primarily used to shape the body, which we will briefly address below, and which might require yet another concept, $drug_4$. As we will see in the next sections, it is common for substances to shift between $drug_1$ and $drug_3$ status, depending on how influential groups in society think of them, particularly lawmakers and those in the medical world.

Classification Systems

We can now compare this theoretical summary with the way the authorities deal with drugs practically: In the US, for example, the Controlled Substances Act of 1971 distinguishes five categories in Schedule I to V. Those substances included in the first are considered to have a high potential for "abuse", but without being of medical use, at least not according to the general opinion in medicine. Schedule II substances are perceived as similarly dangerous, because of their potential to lead to severe psychological and physical dependence, but are also accepted for their therapeutic applications. The prescription stimulants we addressed in so much detail previously fall into this category. Schedules III to V are then increasingly viewed as less harmful.

Many other countries have enacted a similar system, reflecting the same rationale, such as the one established by the Misuse of Drugs Act of 1971 in the United Kingdom, which calls the levels "Schedules 1 to 5" and distinguishes substances into Classes A, B, and C. The similarities between these two and many more countries around the world are no coincidence. International treaties, especially the Single Convention on Narcotic Drugs of 1961, the Convention on Psychotropic Substances of 1971, and the Convention Against Illicit Traffic in Narcotic Drugs and Psychotropic Substances of 1988, were proliferated through the United Nations, particularly on the initiative of the US. As of 2021, roughly 190 countries have ratified these treaties (International Narcotics Control Board, 2022).

The importance of these treaties should not be underestimated: For example, while this book was being written, the Scientific Service of the German Federal Parliament published a report about the obstacles associated with legalizing cannabis, one of the major projects of the present governing coalition of Social Democrats, Greens, and Liberals. That the European Union independently ratified these treaties poses, according to the report, a serious problem to the planned legalization.[1] Meanwhile, researchers keep criticizing—some of them harshly—the status quo as

[1] "Vorgaben des Europäischen Unionsrechts im Hinblick auf eine mitgliedstaatliche Legalisierung von Cannabis" of August 16, 2022, reference number PE 6–3000 – 043/22, online at: https://www.bundestag.de/ausarbeitungen

arbitrary and unscientific. One of them is the neuropsychopharmacologist David Nutt, with whom we are already familiar as one of the participants in the debate on neuroenhancement in the previous chapter. He and the London-based Independent Scientific Committee on Drugs, now simply called "Drug Science", proposed an alternative account, which is summarized in Box 4.1 (Kupferschmidt, 2014; see also Nutt et al., 2010; van Amsterdam et al., 2015).

This ranking is based on experts' estimations. For the harm to users, shown in Box 4.1, physical (e.g., damage to the body, increased mortality), psychological (e.g., dependence), and social factors (e.g., loss of

---

Box 4.1   An Alternative View on Drug Harms to the Users

Professor David Nutt and the Independent Scientific Committee on Drugs rated drug harms. Their list of 20 selected substances, from the most to the least dangerous, is as follows:

1. Crack cocaine
2. Heroin
3. Crystal meth
4. Alcohol
5. Cocaine
6. Amphetamine (Speed)
7. Gamma-hydroxybutyric acid (GHB)
8. Tobacco
9. Ketamine
10. Benzodiazepine
11. Mephedrone
12. Cannabis
13. Methadone
14. butane
15. MDMA (Ecstasy)
16. Anabolic steroids
17. Khat
18. LSD (Acid)
19. Buprenorphine
20. Magic mushrooms

Table 4.1 Drug Harms and Prison Sentences, UK

Class	Includes	Possession	Dealing
A	Ecstasy, LSD, heroin, cocaine, crack, magic mushrooms,	7 years	Life amphetamines (injected)
B	Amphetamines, cannabis, Ritalin, ketamine	5 years	14 years
C	Tranquilizers, some painkillers, GHB	2 years	14 years

Description: Substances as classified by the UK Misuse of Drugs Act, from Class A (most dangerous) to Class C (least dangerous), and the maximum prison sentences for possession and dealing. Source: Nutt (2020)

relationships) were quantified (see Nutt et al., 2010). Notice the stark contrast to the legal classification in the UK (Table 4.1). A similar ranking of the harm to others rated aspects such as injury, crime, or family adversities.

This way of looking at drugs is not without critique, from both within science and by nonscientists. For example, it has been argued, in my view with at least some justification, that alcohol or tobacco look so extremely negative on this assessment due to the high prevalence of their use and that it also makes no sense to compare freely available and strictly prohibited substances in this way (see Caulkins et al., 2011). Caulkins and colleagues also suggested that these experts' estimations might be biased by the fact that they see disproportionally many severe cases of substance use because of their clinical work as medical doctors. We have also discussed in Chap. 2 that the risk of addiction is a characteristic not only of the consumers and the substance but also of the environment they live in. For this reason, I have refrained from showing the results of the—in my view, somewhat arbitrary—ratings of social harm.

Nevertheless, Nutt and colleagues developed and keep developing a science-based alternative view on drugs. Even if their model is pragmatic and does not represent "the whole truth", it emphasizes that the official stance of the drug authorities is at least somewhat arbitrary and inconsistent. That alcohol and tobacco appear to be so dangerous to the users is in stark contrast to the legally enforced classification of drug harms. Alcohol, fourth on the scientists' list (Box 4.1), is regulated such that it may not be made available to minors, but can be bought by adults more or less freely in most countries; by contrast, amphetamine (Speed) and similar stimulants, strictly regulated as Schedule II substances in many countries and even absolutely prohibited in some, are regularly prescribed to children

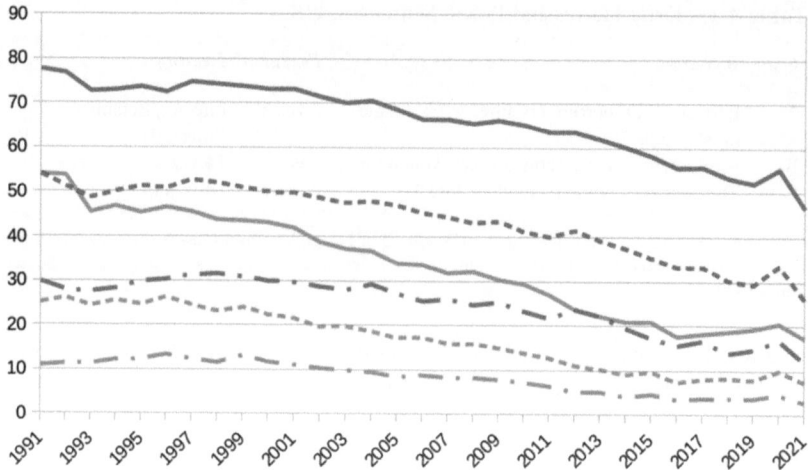

Fig. 4.1 Alcohol Use Among 8th and 12th Graders in the US. Prevalence (in percent) of alcohol use among 8th (green) and 12th graders (red) in the US. The prevalence rates for past year (continuous lines), past month (dashed lines), and binge drinking (dashed with dots) are shown. Binge drinking was defined as five or more drinks in a row during the last two weeks. Source: Monitoring the Future (Miech et al., 2022)

with an ADHD diagnosis in the US, and actually even more commonly to very young children aged 5–12 than those aged 13–17 (Anderson, 2018). Yet, if they later obtain the same substances as adults without a doctor's prescription, it may be called a felony and lead to a severe prison sentence.

Some might be shocked to read that in Germany, where I grew up, adolescents aged 14 or 15 may still drink beer and wine in public under supervision of their parents (§9 *Jugendschutzgesetz*, Protection of Young Persons Act). This is described by some as establishing a predisposition for dependence later in life (Schaller et al., 2017), by others as a way to learn responsible use. Probably both sides have a point. However, a comparison with the prevalence of alcohol use and even binge drinking among 8th and 12th graders in the US (Fig. 4.1), where this is illegal in virtually all jurisdictions, questions the meaningfulness of prohibitive arguments. This is even more so, as alcohol consumption has been decreasing for decades in most countries, including the very permissive Germany (Schaller et al., 2017).

We will return to a discussion of possible implications for drug policy in the book's general conclusion in Chap. 5. For the purpose of the present section, we may conclude that the classification systems authorities use in most countries to regulate substance use neither reflect scientific models nor their citizens' behavior. A more specific example of the scientists' critique is provided by David Nutt, who was dismissed from his function as chair of the British Advisory Council on the Misuse of Drugs after comparing the risk of MDMA (Ecstasy) use with that of horse riding—concluding that the latter led to more adverse events (Nutt, 2009). In a later comparison of cocaine and tobacco use in the UK, he concluded that tobacco was much more physically harmful and addictive (Nutt, 2012). For example, while there were 10 times more tobacco than cocaine users in the UK, 400 times (!) as many deaths per year were related to the former. Nevertheless, he also noted that the possible social harms of cocaine—such as poverty, risk-taking, and antisocial behavior—were higher than for tobacco.

The coronavirus pandemic provided unprecedented insights into how social disruption—unlike war zones such as the Vietnam War discussed before—affects people's substance use in their domestic countries. In Fig. 4.1, we already saw a dip in alcohol use in 2021, most plausibly explained by the fact that this substance is commonly consumed at social events, of which fewer were possible due to measures to reduce the spread of the virus. The same can be seen for other "party drugs" such as MDMA (Ecstasy) or, as we saw in the previous chapter, amphetamine (Speed). However, while alcohol was consumed less on average, the prevalence of high-intensity use (having more than ten drinks in a row in the past weeks) among young adults was the highest measured since 2005 (Patrick et al., 2022). In this age group, cannabis and hallucinogen use reached the highest level recorded since 1988, and cigarette smoking and opioid use reached historical lows (ibid.). While the *average* use thus dropped in nationwide representative surveys, there might thus have been more *individuals* with problematic consumption patterns. This could be an indication that some people use drugs—in the sense of $drug_2$—to cope with their psychological problems. More on this below.

We started this section with a reflection on the meaning of the term "drug" and distinguished in particular two uses, $drug_1$ (approved medical drugs) and $drug_3$ (illicit drugs), which are related to the regulation of substances by the authorities. However, we then also saw how the common classification system is criticized by scientists and that there is a considerable number of minors and adults making their own decisions. These are not necessarily those intended by the official rules. We have thus far already addressed some cultural and historical variability in drug policy. Discussing a few telling historical cases in more detail in the next section will help us to better understand the origins of the way we think about substance use today.

4.2   Historical Examples

We addressed alcohol above to illustrate cultural differences in how substances are perceived. This psychoactive organic chemical compound is naturally produced through the fermentation—one might say "digestion"—of sugars by yeasts. It thus occurs in the wild, even without humans producing it, and many animals have been observed consuming it. For example, the pen-tailed treeshrew (*Ptilocercus lowii*) from Malaysia has been found to drink the fermented nectar of palm trees on a daily basis, which can contain up to 3.8% alcohol, comparable to light beer (Wiens et al., 2008). In human history, alcohol production may have already existed more than 13,000 years ago (Wadley & Hayden, 2015).

As the temperance movement against alcohol and other substances gained momentum around 1900, there were actually debates about whether alcohol was a food or not (see Blair, 1888; Levine, 2006; Tupper, 2012). This may not be so surprising when one considers two historical cultural facts: Firstly, without access to clean drinking water, it was sometimes safer to drink (often diluted) beer or wine, even for children, as the alcohol in them killed germs. Secondly, during Christian fasting periods, it was still allowed to consume beverages, as they were fluid, and they were useful because they nourished the body (Levine, 2006; Schivelbusch, 2010; Spode, 1993). In particular, monks often had to do hard work that required some exertion of energy. This could be provided by beer, which is, after all, produced from grains and high in calories. Many monasteries are still famous today for their breweries.

Being able to afford alcoholic beverages was also a status symbol for citizens, while the poor or ascetics drank potentially polluted water from the wells. Even today, in some Mediterranean countries red wine is perceived as part of a meal rather than considered a psychoactive drug (Spode, 2010). In states with a majority of Muslims, by contrast, alcohol is generally forbidden and its consumption is low to virtually nonexistent. But the historical background is complex: Some schools interpret their religious scriptures as only disallowing prayer or attending service when intoxicated, while others ban it (and gambling) altogether as sinful, while yet other schools think that the prohibition only refers to alcohol made from grapes or dates (Michalak & Trocki, 2006; Ruthven, 2012).

While temperance movements existed in many Western countries around 1900, nowhere else did they become as powerful as in the US, finally leading to a constitutional amendment establishing Prohibition in 1920. Scholars have argued that alcohol was a catalyst for an ongoing culture clash when "native born, middle-class non-urban Protestants [...] felt threatened by the working-class, Catholic immigrants who were filling up America's cities during industrialization" (Reinarman, 1994, p. 93; see also Levine, 1984). In this view, society was split "between an 'uptown' that reflected the established Anglo-Saxon culture, typically centred on Sunday attendance at the church, and a 'downtown' community of more recent immigrant groups—Italian, Irish, German—whose most visible expression was the crowded tavern on Saturday night" (Jay, 2010, p. 160). Debates about the substance were highly moralized and particularly focused on the values of self-control and productivity. Medicalizing alcohol use by calling it an "addiction", and thus perceiving it as a major threat to self-control, also occurred in this period and was used as an argument to prohibit the substance (Levine, 1978).

Efforts to move it from drug$_2$ to drug$_3$ status were not entirely successful, though, as there were exemptions for religious use—alcohol has a ritual meaning in Christianity and Judaism—and doctors could prescribe "medical liquor" as well (Gitlin, 2010; Okrent, 2010). This not only provided doctors and pharmacists with extra income but also attracted thieves and forgers who would steal or fake the special prescription forms. In general, alcohol production and distribution was taken over by criminals (see Jay, 2010; Okrent, 2010). Instead of paying taxes, they used the money to bribe police officers. Ultimately, the prices on the black market increased considerably, while the quality and safety of the alcoholic beverages decreased, as they sometimes contained the harmful methanol. In addition to administrative, health- and crime-related problems, as well as the fact that the law became increasingly unpopular, the Great Depression contributed to the failure of Prohibition and its repeal in 1933. As other revenues plunged, the government needed income from tax on alcohol. Reminiscent of this financial rationale and while this book was being written, the Japanese National Tax Agency launched the campaign "Sake Viva!" for people aged between 20 and 39 to develop business ideas to make their peers drink more—and thus increase the government's tax income.[2]

The example of alcohol illustrates several important points: The way people think about substances and their use can be morally loaded. Some researchers have even characterized this period in the US as "temperance and prohibition crusades" (Levine, 1984, 2006; Reinarman, 1994). In Chap. 2, we discussed the example of tranquilizers, used to deal with initiatives against racial discrimination on the assumption that protesters were suffering from schizophrenia. According to the explanations discussed in this section, here we see an inverted case, where substance use is regulated (i.e., criminalized) to deal with social differences, on the assumption that a particular group was prone to addiction and morally inferior. We also saw how complex it was to prohibit an already common psychoactive substance. The next examples, in contrast to domestic alcohol, concern drugs that were imported from abroad.

Cocaine and Opium

When cocaine—a stimulant drug extracted from coca leaf and domestic to South America—was introduced to Europe in the late nineteenth century, it sparked immediate interest among physicians and researchers. For example, a certain Theodor Aschenbrandt, assistant at the department of pharmacology in Würzburg, Germany, and a military surgeon, is reported to have given the substance to Bavarian soldiers during a maneuver in 1883 (Holmstedt & Fredga, 1981). According to him, the soldiers, who had not been informed about their participation in the "experiment", better endured hunger, strain, fatigue, and heavy burdens under the influence of the drug.

An enthusiastic report, probably written by Aschenbrandt himself, is believed to have inspired the young Sigmund Freud (1856–1939), then working as a physician in Vienna, also to experiment with cocaine (ibid.). Freud hypothesized that he could treat opium dependence with the stimulant, but these attempts failed and seriously damaged his reputation because he neglected cocaine's own addictive potential (Bernfeld, 1953; Freud, 1884). However, he and some of his medical colleagues had noticed that the drug numbed their tongues when they consumed it orally, diluted in water. This in turn enabled one of Freud's colleagues, the oph-thalmologist Carl Koller (1857–1944), to make medical history: He applied the substance as the world's first local anesthetic to make once-dreaded eye surgery much more comfortable for the patients (Grinspoon & Bakalar, 1981).

But times change. While the substance was once considered a medical breakthrough and easily available as tincture in pharmacies, as "cocaine wine", or even as Coca Cola to treat a variety of common ailments or sim-ply for enjoyment, it is presently considered a Class A substance under the UK Misuse of Drugs Act, thus one of the drugs deemed *most dangerous*. However, this does not prevent many European citizens (just as people elsewhere) from consuming it. Quite the opposite, as tons of cocaine are smuggled through the harbors of Antwerp or Rotterdam in huge contain-ers every year, to name just one familiar route the drug takes to its many users around the world.

A culturally even more interesting case is opium, made from the seed capsules of the opium poppy (*Papaver somniferum*). We briefly addressed *Opium, the Demon Flower* in Chap. 2, a book popular in the 1920s and beyond, which disseminated demonstrably wrong information about drug users and addiction (Graham-Mulhall, 1926). But let us go back to the nineteenth century first, to the colonial past. The British Empire imported a lot of tea from China, but could not offer similarly interesting goods to the Chinese in return. Paying for the tea—also a stimulant, a drug$_2$—with silver meant a huge trade deficit for Britain (see Jay, 2010).

The colonialists' convenient "solution" consisted in delivering opium, mostly from India, with the aid of Dutch merchants, another important colonial power at the time. This psychoactive substance was popular in China, and not just among the rich. Many poor people used it to make their lives more bearable and, sometimes, when they became too desper-ate, also to bring it to an end. The Chinese authorities, however, were against the drug. As a result, the British had to trade with smugglers and thereby risked political tensions. At a time when China was increasingly struggling with floods, famines, and economic problems, British traders (or "drug dealers"?) became keener and approached high officials behind the Emperor's back. This, in turn, provoked a response from Chinese authorities, who eventually ordered the destruction of almost a year's supply of opium on June 17, 1839. The British Empire responded by waging the first Opium War (1839–1842), which was followed by another some years later (1856–1860), this time also supported by France. China lost both times and was forced to open its market to the foreign traders. It also had to cede Hong Kong to the British, which still has ramifications today.

While China was flooded with British/Indian opium, the substance was also used in hundreds of freely available medicines in Western countries (Reinarman, 1994). Reportedly, addiction had not been an issue until campaigns in the US were launched against *smoking* the drug, which was then framed as the "Mongolian vice" (ibid., p. 93). Toward the end of the nineteenth century, opium dens were also called a "Yellow Peril" (Jay, 2010, p. 153) and racist rumors described Chinese men as making white women dependent on the drug to exploit them sexually. This happened after the railroads and gold mines had been built by Chinese immigrants, and they increasingly competed with domestic workers in a period of economic depression (Reinarman, 1994). What an irony of history that some of them who were not only using opium tinctures as a medicine but "dared" to smoke the drug for pleasure—which was perceived as "novel and shocking" (Jay, 2010, p. 153)—were stigmatized and criminalized for using a substance forcefully introduced into their culture decades earlier by British traders.

We could discuss other illustrative cases here, such as demonizing "hemp" as "marijuana", a "weed with roots in hell" (Jay, 2010, p. 165), stigmatized in a similar way to the "demon flower" of opium in the early twentieth century (Graham-Mulhall, 1926); how Native Americans' drinking has been framed as a problem by the white majority after teaching them alcohol use in the first place (Holmes & Antell, 2001); how "freebase" became "crack cocaine" and LSD a "threat" to society (Reinarman, 1994). Even coffee and tea have repeatedly featured in "drug scares" in our cultural history (Schivelbusch, 2010; Troyer & Markle, 1994). At present, alcohol is once more becoming a target for researchers who emphasize health risks (Burton & Sheron, 2018), although its consumption has been continuously decreasing in many countries since the 1970s (see, for example, Schaller et al., 2017).

Some scholars have described more generally how class, gender, and race played, and still play, a role in drug policy (see, for example, Denham et al., 2021; Dollar, 2019; Laguna, 2018; Netherland & Hansen, 2016; Tiger, 2017). However, our focus here is on substance use, not policy, although we will briefly return to this in the final conclusion. We will complete this section with an example from very recent history and then systematize what we have learned so far, more or less from the book as a whole, in the subsequent section on instrumental use.

A Current Example

While this book was being written, the Dutch government wanted to prohibit another substance nationwide: laughing gas (*nitrous oxide*; see also Box 4.2). It is inhaled by some people, who experience a few moments of euphoria and a change in perception. However, some have complained about the dangers and the nuisance associated with its use. Halfway through 2020, about 90 Dutch municipalities had already taken measures to forbid its recreational use.[3] Sometimes these initiatives covered only parts of their territory, sometimes a whole city or town, and sometimes specifically bars and clubs. In May 2022, the Dutch Ministry of Health, thus the same institution launching the initiative to fight nonmedical stimulant use among students, as we saw in Chap. 3, submitted a request for advice to the State Council (Raad van State) in The Hague. This institution serves not only as the highest administrative court of the country but also as an adviser to the government. While its reports are not strictly binding, they are an indication of how judges will most likely rule on certain issues.

---

[3] "Zo'n 90 gemeenten lopen vooruit op verbod op lachgas, nemen zelf maatregelen", *NOS Nieuws*, July 14, 2020, online at: https://nos.nl/artikel/2340671-zo-n-90-gemeenten-lopen-vooruit-op-verbod-op-lachgas-nemen-zelf-maatregelen

Box 4.2   A Historical Note on Nitrous Oxide

When inhaled, nitrous oxide can lead to an experience of relaxation, euphoria, or audiovisual changes. It was actually well known among intellectuals in the late 19th and early twentieth century. The American philosopher and poet Benjamin P. Blood (1832–1919) became acquainted with it as an anesthetic during a dental operation. In his pamphlet *The Anaesthetic Revelation and the Gist of Philosophy*, he summarized in 34 pages how the gas and other psychoactive substances had opened his mind and enabled him to appreciate the essence of philosophy, "the genius of being" (Blood, 1874, p. 33). This pamphlet was reviewed by none other than the founding father of academic psychology in the US, William James (1842–1910). James, then at the age of 32, "sincerely advise[d] real students of philosophy to write for the pamphlet to its author" and concluded that "[i]t is by no means as important as [Blood] probably believes it, but still thoroughly original and very suggestive."[4]

Several years later, he wrote about the philosophy of Georg W. F. Hegel (1770–1831) in the renowned journal *Mind*, which still exists today and is published by Oxford University Press. In a note to that article, James describes how he "made some observations on the effects of nitrous- oxide-gas-intoxication which have made me understand better than ever before both the strength and the weakness of Hegel's philosophy." The psychologist writes about a "tremendously exciting sense of an intense metaphysical illumination" in which "[t]ruth lies open to the view in depth beneath depth of almost blinding evidence." The gas-induced experience gave him "with unutterable power the conviction that Hegelism was true after all, and that the deepest convictions of my intellect hitherto were wrong" (James, 1882, p. 206).

Another couple of years later, meanwhile at the age of 47, he compared alcohol and nitrous oxide in the article "The Psychology of Belief", again published in *Mind*. James wrote about the former that "[o]ne of the charms of drunkenness unquestionably lies in the

(*continued*)

[4] *The Atlantic Monthly*, November 1874, p. 628.

Box 4.2 (continued)

deepening of the sense of reality and truth which is gained therein." Things would then "seem more utterly what they are, more 'utterly utter' than when we are sober." Referring to Blood's pamphlet, he adds: "This goes to a fully unutterable extreme in the nitrous oxide intoxication, in which a man's very soul will sweat with conviction, and he be all the while unable to tell what he is convinced of at all" (James, 1889, p. 322). *Mind* lists a total of 16 articles containing "nitrous oxide" between 1882 and 1954. A discussion of the veracity of such experiences goes beyond the scope of this book.

The legal initiative would change the Dutch Opium Law (historically dating back to 1919) such that laughing gas would be added to its List II for "soft drugs". This would strictly regulate trade in the substance and require further safety and control measures. However, on July 13, 2022, the State Council concluded that the government had insufficiently justified the prohibition.[5] The Council pointed out that the prohibition would be complex because the substance is commonly used in medicine (e.g., as a painkiller or narcotic) and in preparing foods (especially whipped cream). Such applications—remaining legal under the proposed law—would make the establishment of a prohibition on recreational use alone difficult, and it was questionable whether the additional human resources required to enforce the law would be available. The Council also found that the prohibition in the proposed form might be unconstitutional because it did not sufficiently justify a restriction of free trade in the substance, which is a liberal value in itself.

Although that made the prohibition of nitrous oxide in the Netherlands seem unlikely, the Dutch government announced its ban, effective from January 1, 2023, on November 14, 2022.[6] In the public announcement,

[5] Advice "Wijziging van het Opiumwetbesluit en lijst II…" of July 13, 2022, reference number W13.22.00063/III, online at: https://www.raadvanstate.nl/actueel/nieuws/@131421/w13-22-00063-iii/

[6] https://www.rijksoverheid.nl/actueel/nieuws/2022/11/14/per-1-januari-2023-verbod-op-lachgas

the state secretary of the Ministry for Health referred to the "enormous health risk" of the substance and "terrible accidents" related to its use on the road. In reaction to that decision, representatives of the Dutch nitrous oxide merchants immediately declared to step to the courts to have the prohibition overturned. It is now up to the judges to rule on its legitimacy.

For our purpose, it is interesting to see how the dangers were assessed. A report[7] on behalf of the Ministry of Health stated that the risk for the individual consumer was low to medium, as the substance caused rather mild side effects, such as headache, dizziness, or tingling sensations. These would commonly occur after using 5 to 10 balloons filled with the gas. Poisoning required more than 50 balloons. Damage to public health could be medium to high, insofar as some people experienced paralysis after use, sometimes even serious paraplegia. The mechanism behind this is a reduction in vitamin B_{12}, which can lead to serious damage in the spinal bone marrow; however, this is reported to occur only rarely, after heavy long-term use (Thompson et al., 2015).

The risk of disturbing public order was considered low to medium. On the one hand, nitrous oxide was not associated with an increase in aggression. However, on the other hand, there had been an increase in traffic accidents related to the substance, for example, when drivers filled balloons while driving. Finally, dangers related to organized crime were reported as low, as the substance was readily available through legal means. There were some indications that criminals traded in it, though, as it was financially lucrative.

For the report, 14 experts were asked to quantify these four categories of risk on scales from 0 to 4. Overall, nitrous oxide received an average final score of 6.7 (where 16 would have been the maximum), thus slightly higher than cannabis and somewhat higher than "magic mushrooms" and ketamine (both between 4 and 5 points). In November 2019, the report concluded that, in comparison to an earlier assessment in 2016, the availability of the substance would be high and associated with a lot of nuisance related to trash (i.e., empty containers) and noise in cities, as well as an

---

[7] "Risocobeoordeling lachgas" of the *Coördinatiepunt Assessment en Monitoring nieuwe drugs* of November 2019, reference number V/050324/01/RB, online at: https://www.rivm.nl/sites/default/files/2019-12/risicobeoordelingsrapport%20lachgas%20 20191209%20beveiligd.pdf

increase in serious adverse health effects. Therefore, it recommended that measures should be taken to counter its use.

In agreement with what we learned in the previous chapters about classification in general, but also about schemes to distinguish different kinds of substances in this chapter in particular, we can see that the way a drug is perceived differs and changes: Assessments depend not only on a specific time and location but also on who the users are, how many there are, and the way a substance is used. "Drug scares" have been documented for centuries, and substances that were once perceived as medically useful, perhaps even as a breakthrough in patient welfare, such as cocaine and opium, may later be perceived as extremely dangerous.

These decisions are often pragmatic and reflect social constructs, not only the intrinsic properties of a substance. An important reference point for such decisions is the availability of alternatives serving similar medical needs but at lower cost or with a better profile of side effects. Thus, opium was replaced by synthetic painkillers such as Aspirin (*acetylsalicylic acid*) or stronger synthetic opioids. These opioids, however, are currently being used in pandemic proportions in the US, leading to tens of thousands of premature deaths annually, to which we will return in Chap. 5. For our present purpose, we can conclude that the substances people consume and what powerful groups in society think about this continuously changes. In the process, it is not uncommon for a $drug_2$ (psychoactive substance) to shift between $drug_1$ (medicine) and $drug_3$ (illicit drug), subject to the various factors we identified above. The common ground to all of this is that people use substances for particular reasons, that is, they use them *instrumentally*.

4.3   INSTRUMENTAL USE

One of the most important findings of Chap. 3 was that while leading scholars framed the neuroenhancement debate as about improving cognition or becoming smarter, data from actual users suggested quite a different understanding. Consumers, especially students, took the substances to feel better and be more motivated to do the academic work they were supposed to do—or to cope with stress. This kind of "mood modification" was already discussed and investigated by academics in the 1960s and 1970s, when tranquilizers became popular (see Smart & Fejer, 1972). From this perspective, taking drugs appears to be an *adaptation* to the demands of a certain environment. This has been similarly described for nonmedical prescription stimulant use in the workplace (Sales et al., 2019).

We also addressed examples of what is commonly considered "recreational use", such as that aimed at experiencing euphoria, intensifying feelings, becoming "high", relaxing, or losing weight. Weight loss, related to the effect of some stimulants to reduce hunger, does not sound very "recreational", however, and could better be understood as changing one's body. This usage, in turn, has been discussed by some scholars more broadly as *bodily image and performance enhancement* and also includes the use of anabolic steroids and human growth hormones (Askew & Williams, 2021; Hope et al., 2021).

The common denominator for all of these variants of human—and probably also nonhuman—behavior is that substances are taken for a certain purpose, such as to attain a particular psychological state, to enable some desired behavior, to look a particular way, thus generally to achieve a desired aim. This has been called "drug instrumentalization" or "instrumental drug use" before (Müller, 2020; Müller & Schumann, 2011; Schleim, 2020). Some researchers even argue that substance use—particularly alcohol, caffeine, and tobacco—has played an important role in our biological and cultural evolution (Braidwood et al., 1953; Müller, 2020; Voigt & Katz, 1986; Wadley, 2016; Wadley & Hayden, 2015). For example, ensuring the availability of beer required humans to settle in a certain area and grow cereals. The final product was less perishable than other beverages, had a high nutritional value, and its effects may have served psychosocial needs in a particular cultural context. This question would be interesting to pursue further, but is not essential for our present purpose. After all, it does not follow from the fact that something was common in the past that it is permissible in the present as well. More importantly, we have already presented examples that illustrate how the status of substance use can switch—or rather be switched—back and forth, between normal, medical, and prohibited.

Treatment and enhancement are about instrumental use as well—and even more obviously so. In the former case, a substance is used to achieve or at least approach a state roughly understood as "health", while in the latter the aim is to go even further, beyond normalcy. That the boundaries between these two categories are somewhat blurred—and perhaps even becoming increasingly fuzzy with the extension of "lifestyle medicine" and "lifestyle drugs" (Bodai et al., 2018; Flower, 2004; Gilbert et al., 2000; Rippe, 2013)—is a further reminder not to overstate the importance of these concepts. Nevertheless, essential distinctions used in drug policy have depended and still depend on drawing such boundaries. Speaking of "instrumental substance use" instead, thus even eschewing the complex and difficult notion of "drug", has many advantages. It is a valid superordinate concept which covers a wide range of people's behaviors without, however, communicating moral values. We will address values independently in the final section of this chapter.

First, we illuminate the new conceptual framework by discussing different goals that can be pursued with substances. What follows below should not be misunderstood as a "drug menu". The book is intended only to inform its readers, not to encourage or discourage substance use. More comprehensive summaries of drugs, their effects, and side effects have been published before (e.g., Gage, 2021; Nutt, 2020; von Heyden et al., 2018). It should also be remembered that the way the substances work differs between people and usually depends not only on the dose, but also individual and contextual effects, such as users' expectations and the reactions of other people (see Langlitz et al., 2021; Schleim, 2022a). Particularly when done excessively, substance use will cease to be instrumental and carry higher risks of adverse events and disease.

Instrumentalization Goals

One researcher who has focused on the reasons behind substance use for many years is Christian P. Müller, professor for addiction medicine at the University Hospital Erlangen in Southern Germany. Over the years, he has elaborated an approach called "drug instrumentalization theory" (Müller, 2020; Müller & Schumann, 2011). This allowed me to see cognitive or neuroenhancement in a new and more consistent way, integrated with substance use more generally (Schleim, 2020). Müller emphasizes the systematic and, one could also say, rational way in which many people instrumentalize substances to achieve certain goals. He distinguishes nine reasons, which we will briefly summarize below: (1) improved social interaction, (2) facilitation of sexual behavior, (3) improved cognitive performance/counteracting fatigue, (4) facilitation of recovery/coping with stress, (5) self-medication for psychological problems, (6) sensory curiosity, (7) euphoria, (8) improved physical appearance, and (9) facilitation of spiritual activities.

Importantly, the drugs' effects are also considered dose-dependent, which means that they only enable the desired effects in a certain "dose window", as pharmacologists call it. As we discussed in Chap. 3, there is, in particular, no "more is better" rule. By contrast, when exceeding an optimal amount, the effects of one and the same substance can shift from enhancement to impairment. This is often called the "inverted-u function". For alcohol, for example, it is also hypothesized that lower or higher doses may affect different neurotransmitter systems in the brain, such as *gamma-amino butyric acid* (GABA) or glutamate (see Campbell et al., 2014). But we need not understand such details on the neurobiological level, where basic research is continuing to unravel the workings of even old substances such as alcohol or amphetamine.

Müller writes that alcohol, cannabis, and stimulants (e.g., caffeine, nicotine, cocaine, and the amphetamines, including MDMA/Ecstasy) can improve social interaction. Alcohol, for example, can help people deal with anxiety, discomfort, and inhibition in social contexts, which one might also simply call "shyness". These effects usually require a low dose, while higher amounts are associated with increased impairments. Many of the stimulants are consumed at social events such as festivals or parties, partially to increase arousal and decrease fatigue. However, some of them are associated with aggression as well. Müller also points out that the same substances can facilitate sexual behavior, the second of the nine aims. This seems to be the case for establishing contact with someone, rather than the intercourse itself. After all, some substances can impair sexual functioning, particularly erection in men. Improving sexual behavior or the experience itself has previously been termed "pharmacosex" or "chemsex" (see Moyle et al., 2020).

The third goal is improving cognitive performance, which we discussed extensively in the previous chapter. In line with our conclusion, Müller writes that "there is little evidence for a significant increase in cognitive performance in a healthy individual with full mental capacity after any kind of psychoactive drug" (Müller, 2020, p. 5). However, he also notes that caffeine, nicotine, and other stimulants can compensate cognitive impairment associated with fatigue. This is closely related to the fourth aim: the facilitation of recovery and coping with stress. Here, Müller addresses alcohol, cannabis, cocaine, methamphetamine ("Crystal Meth"), barbiturates, and benzodiazepines. The last two are commonly prescribed for anxiety and sleeping problems.

Drug instrumentalization as self-medication, the fifth goal, is very complex: On the one hand, there is evidence that, as we have discussed above, substances are used to cope with psychological problems such as stress and anxiety, which in turn can be associated with a mental disorder. On the other hand, drug use can itself be a causal factor for mental disorders. Müller in particular discusses alcohol, nicotine, and cannabis—commonly used in many countries—and their relation to depression, post-traumatic stress disorder, and schizophrenia. For example, depression and alcohol dependence are frequently diagnosed together in clinical samples and "[i]n the majority of co-morbid cases, it appears that an established alcohol addiction may induce major depression" (ibid., p. 6). He also addresses the risk that people may eschew more efficient treatment because of self-medication. However, to what extent they use substances to cope with psychological problems below the threshold of clinical significance, how frequently they may take drugs to consciously or unconsciously deal with symptoms of a mental disorder, whether diagnosed or not, and how often the substance use itself causally contributes to the disorder has to be clarified better by further research.

Müller's sixth and ninth aims are, in my view, better discussed together, as they are primarily about hallucinogenic drugs: People may use them to deal with boredom, out of curiosity, novelty seeking, or to have spiritual experiences and insights, as those described by William James (Box 4.2). Substances commonly taken for these purposes are mescaline, psilocybin, LSD, ketamine, GHB, and DMT. Müller points out that cannabis can also be used to "expand environmental and self-perception" and that MDMA "exerts hallucinogenic effects but also induces a unique feeling of 'divine oneness' with the world" (ibid., p. 7). Use of these substances, though, can also lead to risky behaviors or schizophrenia-like psychoses. The seventh aim of experiencing euphoria, hedonia, or a "high", can be facilitated with alcohol, benzodiazepines, cannabis, LSD, and nicotine. The intensity of such states is described as higher with amphetamine, cocaine, heroin, MDMA, methamphetamine, methylphenidate ("Ritalin"), or morphine use.

The final aim, improved physical appearance and attractiveness, can be divided into a desire for a lean body, on the one hand, or a more muscular appearance, on the other. The former is described as more common among women, the latter among men. Stimulants such as amphetamine or cocaine are associated with attenuating hunger and weight loss. By contrast, anabolic steroids are used to gain more muscle mass (see Askew & Williams, 2021; Hope et al., 2021). Müller points out that steroids might also directly improve self-esteem and self-confidence, and not only indirectly through consumers' increased satisfaction with their bodies (Müller, 2020).

Theoretical Reflection

Merely describing these possible uses implies neither endorsing nor disapproving of them. Elsewhere, I suggested that Müller's nine categories could be reduced to four: (1) psychological activation/enhancement, (2) psychological dampening/relaxation, (3) new experiences, and (4) body shaping (Schleim, 2022b). Müller's more comprehensive list has the advantage of illustrating more practical examples of instrumental substance use. I would argue that my condensed categorization allows us to better understand the psychology behind it. The first two amount to obtaining more of a desired psychological state or process (e.g., more attention) or less of an undesired one (e.g., anxiety). The third is orthogonal to this positive/negative distinction in two ways, as psychedelic experiences do not merely offer a greater or lesser sense of what is present, but something genuinely new—and this can be perceived as positive (e.g., "new insights" about oneself) or negative (e.g., a "horror trip"). Finally, changing one's physical appearance is different from changing one's psychological processes.

Yet, as has been emphasized so often in the book already, we should not overvalue the meaning of this conceptual distinction. After all, *less* fatigue could also mean *more* attention, and vice versa; gaining new insights might make one feel happier or depressed; feeling better might enable one to live in a healthier way, which could also improve one's physical appearance; and having the leaner or more muscular body one desires so much may increase one's satisfaction and self-confidence. But merely saying that the psychological and physiological domains, or that enhancement and impairment are related—that more or less everything is associated with anything—would not increase our understanding. The nine, or only four categories, are thus, once more, a pragmatic way to make sense of something, in this case substance use. How we perceive it also depends on the perspective we take.

Those readers who are already primarily informed about drug harms might find it difficult to accept the notion of instrumental substance use. However, repeating a question from the previous chapter: *Why would users use the substances, if that's of no use?* Others may recognize their own consumption patterns in the goals described above. However, for yet others it might just be a confirmation of what they have long known about drugs. It goes without saying that substance use may have unwanted side effects, but the same holds for medical drugs and—depending on the amount ingested—even beverages and food. In his conclusion, Müller emphasizes again the importance of finding the right dose window for instrumental use to keep benefits and risks in a reasonable balance (Müller, 2020). In line with what we have argued in Chap. 2, only a minority of substance users become addicted, while those engaging in instrumental consumption can use checklists to identify problematic patterns.

Müller also addresses the risk of overinstrumentalization: Imagine someone drinking alcohol or smoking cannabis in the evening to deal with work-related stress. This substance use may help the person to relax and in turn to feel and work better the next day. However, if they then increase their workload knowing that the unwanted effects can be dealt with, the amount of stress might increase, which may in turn require the person to consume more of the substance to gain the desired result. Higher doses increase the risks of adaptation, dependence, side effects, and disease. This illustrates the reasonable boundaries of instrumental substance use and also the biopsychosocial context in which it occurs, with someone's decision (psychology) having repercussions on the body (biology) and circumstances (society), which all interact with each other.

While some scholars see instrumental substance use as a part of human nature and welcome opportunities to make more of one's life (e.g., Miller, 2011), others point to the risk of excessive individualization (e.g., Schleim, 2014; Wu, 2011). Imagine that employers coerce employees to use substances in order to increase performance in an already-highly productive and competitive context. David Nutt mentioned a real example from the Soviet era, where stimulant drugs were used in factories to enhance workers' output (Nutt, 2020). Increased competition among truck drivers during America's "first amphetamine epidemic", as Nicolas Rasmussen called it, may be another example (Rasmussen, 2008). This reminds us of the puzzle posed at the beginning of Chap. 3: At an already-enhanced level, the same question of whether even higher performance would be better comes up again. Instrumental substance use can thus get us only so far. At some point, we would have to concede a limit to prevent serious damage to body and mind. These thoughts anticipate the discussion of values in the final section of this chapter.

4.4   VALUES

Thus far, we have focused on understanding the problems, the scholarly debate, and the scientific facts related to health, mental health, enhancement, and substance use. In Chap. 3, we saw that issues concerning safety, coercion, and fairness have been frequently addressed by ethicists. However, merely describing these does not answer the question of whether instrumental substance use should be generally permissible in society or whether one should do it. Even a logical or mathematical proof depends on the axioms and assumptions one makes. In ethical matters, we have to deal with even less certainty. What provides us with some guidance is the identification of different positions and values that are relevant to our present topic. One source of information is a closely related academic debate that occurred in the 1970s, decades before scholars began talking about "neuroenhancement" or "instrumental substance use".[8]

American psychiatrist Gerald Klerman (1928–1992), who was a professor at Harvard University and later director of a prominent drug prevention program under US president Jimmy Carter, suggested several useful terms in the discussion, opposing "psychotropic hedonism" to "pharmacological Calvinism" (Klerman, 1970, 1972). The latter reflects the Protestant work ethic, which can be summarized as "No pain, no gain". Psychotropic hedonism, by contrast, focuses on the now: "Why wait when I can fulfill my needs and achieve my goals now, if necessary, by pharmacological means?"

At the time, however, the renowned American medical ethicist Robert M. Veatch (1939–2020), who would later become professor at Georgetown University in Washington, D.C. and researcher at the Kennedy Institute of Ethics, criticized Klerman's explanation as being overly simplistic (Veatch, 1977). Drawing on Max Weber's (1864–1920) analysis of the Protestant work ethic (Weber, 1905), he concluded that substance use to increase efficiency could be permissible from a Christian perspective. However, advocates of an ethic that is based on the "wisdom of nature" and is critical of artificial interventions into the body would be particularly opposed to this.

---

[8] The following paragraphs on Klerman and Veach are adapted from my report on brain doping (Schleim, 2022b), which can be accessed online at: https://doi.org/10.33612/227882920

Klerman's psychotropic hedonism most closely corresponds to what Veatch called a "Protean ethic", which is named after Proteus, the Greek god of rivers and oceanic bodies of water, who was able to change his form. In this view, substances are used to perpetually change and to adapt to external demands. Proponents of this ethic deny the existence of a permanent essence of human beings. Today, these ideas from the 1970s resemble precursors of globalization, competitive pressure, and life-long learning. Klerman and Veatch did agree on one thing, however—that social values are articulated in the way people treat substances. These values, according to Klerman, create divisions between different social groups: the old and the young, the more and the less educated, the poor and the rich, and groups with different religious or cultural backgrounds (Klerman, 1970). Here, the psychiatrist lamented that they lacked a suitable word for nonmedical substance use:

> In our society there is no suitable label for the use of drugs to enhance pleasure or performance. It is sometimes called social drug use, but this term is not part of our scientific lexicon. [...] The fact that we don't have an established nomenclature for nontherapeutic drug use is in itself an indication of society's conflict. (Klerman, 1970, p. 316)

In this respect, times have changed. As we have seen in Chap. 3, "cognitive" and "neuroenhancement" became popular terms in the early 2000s. However, according to the discussion in the present chapter, "instrumental substance use" would be a better alternative. Several goals were addressed in the previous section. Earlier in the book, we also found that distinctions between diseases/disorders, health/normalcy, and enhancement remain vague, even if there are many cases that can be assigned unambiguously to only one of the categories. But *if* health is now understood as the ability to adapt and to self-manage (Huber et al., 2011), *if* renowned professors advising governments emphasize the importance of maximizing one's "mental capital" (Beddington et al., 2008), *if* other professors from elite universities call the consumption of legally prohibited stimulants to improve one's cognitive performance "responsible use" under certain conditions (Greely et al., 2008), and *if* many people are using substances instrumentally anyway, how much sense does it make to prohibit and criminalize this behavior?

Indeed, in line with the Protean ethic, some scholars have described instrumental substance use as "self-improvement" (Askew & Williams,

2021) or "competitive entrepreneurialism" in the context of "neoliberalism" (Mann, 2021). Miller and Müller wholeheartedly welcomed the possibilities of using substances to adapt to the demands of a certain environment (Miller, 2011; Müller, 2020; Müller & Schumann, 2011). But should adaptation be limitless? How far might coercion go before too much *autonomy* (literally, having one's own laws) is lost and *heteronomy* (having others' laws) reigns? Aren't we already very productive and isn't this high level of productivity already causing severe damage to life and the environment on planet earth? Doesn't Wu have a point when he emphasizes the risks of too much individualization (Wu, 2011)? And isn't Inon's critique valid when he points out that people's emotional responses in competitive environments also tell us something about these environments, not just the people (Inon, 2019)?

The argument from the perspective of evolution suggested that instrumental substance use was common and normal, probably even advantageous in our past (Braidwood et al., 1953; Voigt & Katz, 1986; Wadley, 2016; Wadley & Hayden, 2015). But it does not follow from this alone that it is still morally the right thing to do in the present and future. There is also an essential difference between an adaptation that increases the chances of survival in the face of natural hardship and one that is a response to unequal human-made social structures. In the latter case, the debate also needs to address the political foundations of living together. That the pressure to engage in instrumental substance use is particularly strong under the extraordinary conditions found in professional sports and warfare (see Nutt, 2020) also raises the question of whether this is the right model for society at large.

In times of peace and when survival is not at risk, other values—such as autonomy, distributive justice, social participation, and sustainability—should at least be considered alongside performance enhancement. Above all, we should also recall that cognitive improvement might have a lower priority in society at large than it does among professors in scholarly debates (Schleim, 2014). As we have seen in Chap. 3, even their own students seem to think differently about the importance of substance use to enhance performance.

References

Anderson, J. (2018). Statistical Brief #514: Reported Diagnosis and Prescription Utilization Related to Attention Deficit Hyperactivity Disorder in Children Ages 5–17, 2008–2015. *Medical Expenditure Panel Survey*, August 2018. https://meps.ahrq.gov/data_files/publications/st514/stat514.pdf.

Askew, R., & Williams, L. (2021). Rethinking enhancement substance use: A critical discourse studies approach. *The International Journal on Drug Policy*, *95*, 102994.

Beddington, J., Cooper, C. L., Field, J., Goswami, U., Huppert, F. A., Jenkins, R., Jones, H. S., Kirkwood, T. B., Sahakian, B. J., & Thomas, S. M. (2008). The mental wealth of nations. *Nature*, *455*, 1057–1060.

Bernfeld, S. (1953). Freud's studies on cocaine, 1884–1887. *Journal of the American Psychoanalytic Association*, *1*, 581–613.

Blair, H. W. (1888). *The temperance movement: Or, the conflict between man and alcohol*. W. E. Smythe.

Blood, B. P. (1874). *The anaesthetic revelation and the gist of philosophy*. N.D..

Bodai, B. I., Nakata, T. E., Wong, W. T., Clark, D. R., Lawenda, S., Tsou, C., Liu, R., Shiue, L., Cooper, N., Rehbein, M., Ha, B. P., & Campbell, T. M. (2018). Lifestyle medicine: A brief review of its dramatic impact on health and survival. *The Permanente Journal*, *22*, 17–25.

Braidwood, R. J., Sauer, J. D., Helbaek, H., Mangelsdorf, P. C., Cutler, H. C., Coon, C. S., Coon, C. S., Linton, R., Steward, J., & Oppenheim, A. L. (1953). Did man once live by beer alone? *American Anthropologist*, *55*, 515–526.

Burton, R., & Sheron, N. (2018). No level of alcohol consumption improves health. *The Lancet*, *392*, 987–988.

Campbell, A. E., Sumner, P., Singh, K. D., & Muthukumaraswamy, S. D. (2014). Acute effects of alcohol on stimulus-induced gamma oscillations in human primary visual and motor cortices. *Neuropsychopharmacology*, *39*, 2104–2113.

Caulkins, J. P., Reuter, P., & Coulson, C. (2011). Basing drug scheduling decisions on scientific ranking of harmfulness: False promise from false premises. *Addiction*, *106*, 1886–1890.

Denham, B., Cacciatore, S., & Caves, M. (2021). Bleeding Borders and enemies within: How newsmagazine covers portrayed drugs of abuse, 1979–2019. *Contemporary Drug Problems*, *48*, 3–18.

Dollar, C. B. (2019). Criminalization and drug "wars" or medicalization and health "epidemics": How race, class, and neoliberal politics influence drug Laws. *Critical Criminology*, *27*, 305–327.

Flower, R. (2004). Lifestyle drugs: Pharmacology and the social agenda. *Trends in Pharmacological Sciences*, *25*, 182–185.

Freud, S. (1884). Ueber coca. *Centralblatt für die gesammte Therapie*, *2*, 289–314.

Gage, S. (2021). *Say why to drugs: Everything you need to know about the drugs we take and why we get high*. Hodder Education.

Gilbert, D., Walley, T., & New, B. (2000). Lifestyle medicines. *BMJ*, *321*(7272), 1341–1344.

Gitlin, M. (2010). *The prohibition era.* ABDO Pub.

Goodman, J., Lovejoy, P. E., & Sherratt, A. (2007). *Consuming habits: Global and historical perspectives on how cultures define drugs* (2nd ed.). Routledge.

Graham-Mulhall, S. (1926). *Opium, the demon Flower.* Montrose Publishing Co.

Greely, H., Sahakian, B., Harris, J., Kessler, R. C., Gazzaniga, M., Campbell, P., & Farah, M. J. (2008). Towards responsible use of cognitive-enhancing drugs by the healthy. *Nature, 456,* 702–705.

Grinspoon, L., & Bakalar, J. B. (1981). Coca and cocaine as medicines: An historical review. *Journal of Ethnopharmacology, 3,* 149–159.

Hengartner, T., & Merki, C. M. (Eds.) (1999). Genussmittel: ein kulturgeschichtliches Handbuch. Frankfurt am Main: Campus Verlag.

Holmes, M. D., & Antell, J. A. (2001). The social construction of American Indian drinking: Perceptions of American Indian and white officials. *The Sociological Quarterly, 42,* 151–173.

Holmstedt, B., & Fredga, A. (1981). Sundry episodes in the history of coca and cocaine. *Journal of Ethnopharmacology, 3,* 113–147.

Hope, V. D., Underwood, M., Mulrooney, K., Mazanov, J., van de Ven, K., & McVeigh, J. (2021). Human enhancement drugs: Emerging issues and responses. *International Journal of Drug Policy, 95,* 103459.

Huber, M., Knottnerus, J. A., Green, L., Van Der Horst, H., Jadad, A. R., Kromhout, D., Leonard, B., Lorig, K., Van Loureiro, M. I., & der Meer, J. W. (2011). How should we define health? *BMJ, 343,* d4163.

Inon, M. (2019). Fooled by 'smart drugs'—Why shouldn't pharmacological cognitive enhancement be liberally used in education? *Ethics and Education, 14,* 54–69.

International Narcotics Control Board. (2022). *Report of the international narcotics control board for 2021.* United Nations.

James, W. (1882). On Some Hegelisms. *Mind, 7,* 186–208.

James, W. (1889). The psychology of belief. *Mind, 14,* 321–352.

Jay, M. (2010). *High society: The central role of mind-altering drugs in history, science and culture.* Park Street Press.

Klerman, G. L. (1970). Drugs and social values. *International Journal of the Addictions, 5,* 313–319.

Klerman, G. L. (1972). Psychotropic hedonism vs. pharmacological Calvinism. *The Hastings Center Report, 2,* 1–3.

Kupferschmidt, K. (2014). The dangerous professor. *Science, 343,* 478–481.

Laguna, S. (2018). Constructing drug using victims: Race and class in policy debates on ecstasy use in the U.S. *Contemporary Drug Problems, 45,* 67–81.

Langlitz, N., Dyck, E., Scheidegger, M., & Repantis, D. (2021). Moral psychopharmacology needs moral inquiry: The case of psychedelics. *Frontiers in Psychiatry, 12,* 680064.

Levine, H. G. (1978). The discovery of addiction. Changing conceptions of habitual drunkenness in America. *Journal of Studies on Alcohol, 39,* 143–174.

Levine, H. G. (1984). The alcohol problem in America: From temperance to alcoholism. *British Journal of Addiction, 79,* 109–119.

Levine, H. G. (2006). Drunkenness and Civilization. In R. Behr, H. Cremer-Schäfer & S. Scheerer (Eds.), *Kriminalitäts-Geschichten, Hamburger Studien zur Kriminologie und Kriminalpolitik, Band 41* (pp. 133–156). Hamburg: Lit Verlag.

Mann, J. (2021). Cognitive enhancing drug use by students in the context of neoliberalism: Cheating? Or, a legitimate expression of competitive entrepreneurialism? *The International Journal on Drug Policy, 95,* 102907.

Michalak, L., & Trocki, K. (2006). Alcohol and Islam: An overview. *Contemporary Drug Problems, 33,* 523–562.

Miech, R. A., Johnston, L. D., O'Malley, P. M., Bachman, J. G., Schulenberg, J. E., & Patrick, M. E. (2022). *Monitoring the future national survey results on drug use, 1975–2021: Volume I, secondary school students.* Institute for Social Research, The University of Michigan.

Miller, G. F. (2011). Optimal drug use and rational drug policy. *Behavioral and Brain Sciences, 34,* 318–319.

Moyle, L., Dymock, A., Aldridge, A., & Mechen, B. (2020). Pharmacosex: Reimagining sex, drugs and enhancement. *International Journal of Drug Policy, 86,* 102943.

Müller, C. P. (2020). Drug instrumentalization. *Behavioural Brain Research, 390,* 112672.

Müller, C. P., & Schumann, G. (2011). Drugs as instruments: A new framework for non-addictive psychoactive drug use. *Behavioral and Brain Sciences, 34,* 293–310.

Netherland, J. & Hansen, H. B. (2016). The War on Drugs That Wasn't: Wasted Whiteness, "Dirty Doctors," and Race in Media Coverage of Prescription Opioid Misuse. Culture, Medicine, and Psychiatry, 40, 664–686.

Ng, Q. X., Venkatanarayanan, N., & Ho, C. Y. (2017). Clinical use of Hypericum perforatum (St John's wort) in depression: A meta-analysis. *Journal of Affective Disorders, 210,* 211–221.

Nutt, D. J. (2009). Equasy—An overlooked addiction with implications for the current debate on drug harms. *Journal of Psychopharmacology, 23,* 3–5.

Nutt, D. J. (2012). *Drugs—Without the hot air: Minimizing the harms of legal and illegal drugs.* UIT Cambridge.

Nutt, D. J. (2020). *Drugs—Without the hot air: Minimizing the harms of legal and illegal drugs* (2nd ed.). UIT Cambridge.

Nutt, D. J., King, L. A., & Phillips, L. D. (2010). Drug harms in the UK: A multicriteria decision analysis. *The Lancet, 376,* 1558–1565.

Okrent, D. (2010). *Last call: The rise and fall of prohibition.* Scribner.

Parascandola, J. (1995). The drug habit: The association of the word 'drug' with abuse in American history. In R. Porter & M. Teich (Eds.), *Drugs and narcotics in history* (pp. 156–167). Cambridge University Press.

Patrick, M. E., Schulenberg, J. E., Miech, R. A., Johnston, L. D., O'Malley, P. M., & Bachman, J. G. (2022). *Monitoring the future panel study annual report: National data on substance use among adults ages 19 to 60.* Institute for Social Research, The University of Michigan.

Rasmussen, N. (2008). *On speed: The many lives of amphetamine.* New York University Press.

Reinarman, C. (1994). The social construction of drug scares. In P. A. Adler & P. Adler (Eds.), *Constructions of deviance: Social power, context, and interaction* (pp. 92–104). Wadsworth.

Rippe, J. M. (2013). *Lifestyle medicine* (2nd ed.). CRC Press.

Ruthven, M. (2012). *Islam: A very short introduction* (2nd ed.). Oxford University Press.

Sales, P., Murphy, F., Murphy, S., & Lau, N. (2019). Burning the candle at both ends: Motivations for non-medical prescription stimulant use in the American workplace. *Drugs: Education. Prevention and Policy, 26,* 301–308.

Schaller, K., Kahnert, S., & Mons, U. (2017). *Alkoholatlas Deutschland 2017.* Deutsches Krebsforschungszentrum.

Schivelbusch, W. (2010). *Das Paradies, der Geschmack und die Vernunft: eine Geschichte der Genussmittel* (7th ed.). Fischer.

Schleim, S. (2014). Whose well-being? Common conceptions and misconceptions in the enhancement debate. *Frontiers in Systems Neuroscience, 8,* 148.

Schleim, S. (2018). Medications and drugs as social expectations change. In M. Mercer (Ed.), *altered states. Substanzen in der zeitgenössischen Kunst* (pp. 292–303). Kunstpalais.

Schleim, S. (2020). Neuroenhancement as instrumental drug use: Putting the debate in a different frame. *Frontiers in Psychiatry, 11,* 567497.

Schleim, S. (2022a). Grounded in biology: Why the context-dependency of psychedelic drug effects means opportunities, not problems for anthropology and pharmacology. *Frontiers in Psychiatry, 13,* 906487.

Schleim, S. (2022b). *Pharmacological enhancement: The facts and myths about brain doping.* Theory and History of Psychology, University of Groningen.

Smart, R. G., & Fejer, D. (1972). Drug use among adolescents and their parents: Closing the generation gap in mood modification. *Journal of Abnormal Psychology, 79,* 153–160.

Spode, H. (1993). *Die Macht der Trunkenheit: Kultur- und Sozialgeschichte des Alkohols in Deutschland.* Leske + Budrich.

Spode, H. (2010). Trinkkulturen in Europa. Strukturen, Transfers, Verflechtungen. In J. Wienand & C. Wienand (Eds.), *Die kulturelle Integration Europas* (pp. 361–391). VS Verlag für Sozialwissenschaften.

Thompson, A. G., Leite, M. I., Lunn, M. P., & Bennett, D. L. H. (2015). Whippits, nitrous oxide and the dangers of legal highs. *Practical Neurology, 15,* 207–209.

Tiger, R. (2017). Race, class, and the framing of drug epidemics. *Contexts, 16,* 46–51.

Troyer, R. J., & Markle, G. E. (1994). Coffee drinking: An emerging social problem? In P. A. Adler & P. Adler (Eds.), *Constructions of deviance: Social power, context, and interaction* (pp. 73–91). Wadsworth.

Tupper, K. W. (2012). Psychoactive substances and the English language: "Drugs," discourses, and public policy. *Contemporary Drug Problems, 39*, 461–492.

van Amsterdam, J., Nutt, D., Phillips, L., & van den Brink, W. (2015). European rating of drug harms. *Journal of Psychopharmacology, 29*, 655–660.

Veatch, R. M. (1977). Value foundations for drug use. *Journal of Drug Issues, 7*, 253–262.

Voigt, S. H., & Katz, M. M. (1986). Bread and beer: The early use of cereals in the human diet. *Expedition, 28*, 23–34.

von Heyden, M., Jungaberle, H., & Majić, T. (Eds.). (2018). *Handbuch Psychoaktive Substanzen*. Springer.

Wadley, G. (2016). How psychoactive drugs shape human culture: A multidisciplinary perspective. *Brain Research Bulletin, 126*, 138–151.

Wadley, G., & Hayden, B. (2015). Pharmacological influences on the neolithic transition. *Journal of Ethnobiology, 35*(566–584), 519.

Weber, M. (1905). Die protestantische Ethik und der Geist des Kapitalismus (the protestant ethics and the spirit of capitalism). *Archiv für Sozialwissenschaften und Sozialpolitik, XX–XXI*(1–51), 51–110.

Wiens, F., Zitzmann, A., Lachance, M. A., Yegles, M., Pragst, F., Wurst, F. M., von Holst, D., Guan, S. L., & Spanagel, R. (2008). Chronic intake of fermented floral nectar by wild treeshrews. *Proc Natl Acad Sci USA, 105*, 10426–10431.

Wu, K. C.-C. (2011). Governing drug use through neurobiological subject construction: The sad loss of the sociocultural. *Behavioral and Brain Sciences, 34*, 327–328.

CHAPTER 5

Conclusion and Outlook

Abstract The last chapter draws a general conclusion for the whole book with a special emphasis on how, for all major topics (health, enhancement, and substances), definitions matter for how to think about, use, and regulate drugs. The problems of stigmatization and criminalization are addressed together with present challenges for drug policy, such as the opioid epidemic with its high toll of addicted, injured, and even dead people, particularly in the US. The author also presents a personal conclusion on how he himself thinks about drugs and how he instrumentalized substances to write this book.

Keywords Biopower • Opioid epidemic • Drug policy • Harm reduction

> *Ultimately, our drug use is a reflection of our society and should never be considered without the broader context of why healthy people choose to use the drugs in the first place.*
> —Barbara J. Sahakian, professor of clinical neuropsychology at the University of Cambridge, and Sharon Morein-Zamir, associate professor of psychology at Anglia Ruskin University (Sahakian & Morein-Zamir, 2007, p. 1159)

© The Author(s) 2023
S. Schleim, *Mental Health and Enhancement*, Palgrave Studies in Law, Neuroscience, and Human Behavior,
https://doi.org/10.1007/978-3-031-32618-9_5

127

5.1   Overall Conclusion

This book has been a scholarly journey looking at how concepts or definitions interact with things and people. Some of these things were substances called "drugs", while people have been described as "healthy" or "sick", "normal" or "abnormal", or even "disordered". The journey was thus an exemplification of what Ian Hacking called *dynamic nominalism*, the philosophical stance investigating the continuous interaction between a name and that which is named (Hacking, 1999). Hacking, in turn, was inspired by one of Friedrich Nietzsche's (1844–1900) aphorisms from *The Joyous Science*, pointing out that name and essence tend to be confused and that controversies can become increasingly obsessed with names (Nietzsche, 1882/2006). We might also say: At some point there is a risk that classifications or definitions are taken more seriously than that which is being classified or defined. The examples of health (Chap. 1), mental disorders (Chap. 2), enhancement (Chap. 3), or drugs (Chap. 4) all illustrated these features.

We can also make use of the Foucauldian notion of *biopower* to show that these debates are not only happening in the symbolic ivory tower but are actually influencing people's behaviors, bodies, and lives (Foucault, 1976/1978; see also Rose, 2010). After all, advances in neuroscience tempt people to understand their problems as brain problems (see Davis, 2020; Johnson, 2008) and then to act accordingly, for example, by consuming psychoactive substances. We described this behavior as neutrally and broadly as possible as instrumental substance use (Chap. 4). In some contexts, though, such use will be considered a felony and may lead to long prison sentences.

This book is primarily intended as an informative and descriptive, not prescriptive, account. Yet, we must note that the strong emphasis on enhancing performance, even expressed by some governmental authorities (Chap. 3), is in stark contrast to the criminalization and punishment of instrumental substance use aimed at increasing performance in other contexts (Chap. 4). This holds regardless of whether users want to directly improve their cognition or rather do so indirectly by increasing their motivation or counteracting fatigue. Influential scholars have described the "responsible use" of medically regulated or, in some jurisdictions, even completely prohibited stimulants for such purposes (Greely et al., 2008). But decriminalizing such use only in academic or occupational contexts would presume a value judgment such that cognitive performance is more desirable than having fun (so-called recreational use). It can at least be doubted whether the state or legislator should make that judgment for citizens in a politically liberal society. In the meantime, physicians play the role of gatekeeper by sanctioning the instrumental use of stimulants and other psychoactive substances as medically necessary, while the associated diagnoses like ADHD in themselves are controversial (Chap. 2).

A more academically relevant conclusion is that it would be better to discard the concepts of cognitive or neuroenhancement (see also Quednow, 2010; Schleim, 2020, 2022a). This would also have implications for funding decisions and media coverage. While these concepts can—and should, for reasons of consistency and comprehensiveness—be subsumed under instrumental substance use, the enhancement debate has rested on errors from its very inception, as the instrumental use of stimulants as "study drugs" can be documented since at least the 1930s (Anon, 1937; Meerloo, 1937). In particular, the prevalence of their nonmedical use has been *decreasing* since at least the 1980s, use which is framed as cognitive enhancement more plausibly reflects emotional/motivational goals or coping with stress, and the possibilities of pharmaceutical research and practice have been strongly exaggerated (Chap. 3; see also Schleim & Quednow, 2018). This critical stance gains further support from the fact that recent reviews keep reiterating the same questions and identifying ever more layers of complexity, while basic and essential issues about the translation of laboratory findings into real-life settings or the long-term effects of the substances on body and mind remain unanswered even after more than 20 years, not to mention the lack of consensus on ethical and political questions (Dresler et al., 2019; Racine et al., 2021).

5.2   Outlook

As an alternative, present and previous findings on drugs and their effects (see Müller, 2020) should be developed into a comprehensive *instrumental substance use theory* (ISUT). This would allow actual or potential consumers, as well as authorities and legislators, to make better-informed and more consistent decisions, possibly having implications for the lives of hundreds of millions of people around the world. If adaptation, performance, and "entrepreneurial selves" remain highly valued (Fomiatti et al., 2019; Miller, 2011), decriminalizing at least some stimulants should be considered. However, the downside of adaptation, with its individualization and decontextualization of social problems, should also be recognized (Malabou, 2008; Schleim, 2014a; Wu, 2011).

This applies not just to society at large, but to academic settings in particular: Jason Mazanow, for example, wondered why only one in 200 universities had adapted their code of conduct to prohibit the nonmedical use of stimulant drugs (Mazanov, 2019; referring to Aikins et al., 2017). The same goes for the scholarly debate on whether such behavior should be considered as "cheating" (see Greely et al., 2008; Schermer, 2008). While we could reply that, according to our conclusion, that kind of substance use is neither a mass phenomenon nor proven to be efficient in healthy students, a more general answer could point out that these stimulants already *are* strictly regulated by criminal law that naturally applies on campuses as well. Besides that, it is up to educational institutions and their members to discuss stress and performance pressure as well as ways to deal with it. I have been doing so with my own students for more than ten years.

While this book is nearing completion, Biological Psychiatry may be facing a serious crisis now that ever more critical publications are addressing its inability to identify reliable biomarkers for mental disorders or, once again, question the efficacy of the mass prescription of psychopharmacological drugs (see Moncrieff et al., 2022; Schleim, 2022b). When Roger W. Sperry (1913–1994) received the Nobel Prize in Physiology and Medicine in 1981, ten years before the "Decade of the Brain", he suggested that brain researchers should promise practical applications to secure public attention and funds (Sperry, 1981). But if these innovations cannot be realized persistently (see Lewis-Fernandez et al., 2016), this questions the basic assumptions on which a research paradigm is built. Views emphasizing the social causes of psychological distress (Mirowsky & Ross, 2012) may gain momentum. An illustrative example of that is a "Critical Psychiatry" conference presently being prepared in collaboration with scholars from the Vanderbilt University in Nashville, Tennessee, organized by people of different colors and genders, as well as high schoolers, undergrad students, and professors.[1] One of their publicity mottos states: "Engage with history. Pills won't fix what poverty causes."

Another pressing issue remains the opioid epidemic in the US, which has already cost the lives of hundreds of thousands of people. As some scholars argue, it was driven originally by attempts to fight heroin use, the increasing medicalization of pain, socioeconomic problems, and financial

---

[1] https://www.vanderbiltcritpsych.org/

interests within the medical system and pharmaceutic industry (see Nutt, 2020). It became severe when the authorities reduced the availability of the powerful painkillers that were formerly extensively prescribed, with insufficient consideration of the needs of those who had become dependent in the meantime (ibid.). While the "War on Drugs" is commonly justified by the argument that it is aimed at the protection of people, the opioid epidemic provides a counterexample demonstrating that even within the present medical and prohibitive system—and possibly even partially caused by it—consumers' lives are jeopardized (Fig. 5.1).

Scientific views on harm reduction, by contrast, emphasize the important role of prevention, decriminalization, and the treatment of substance use disorders, such as substituting heroin with medically administered methadone (Duff, 2013; Nutt, 2020). Figure 5.1 suggests that, on the one hand, as soon as users become used to a certain substance,

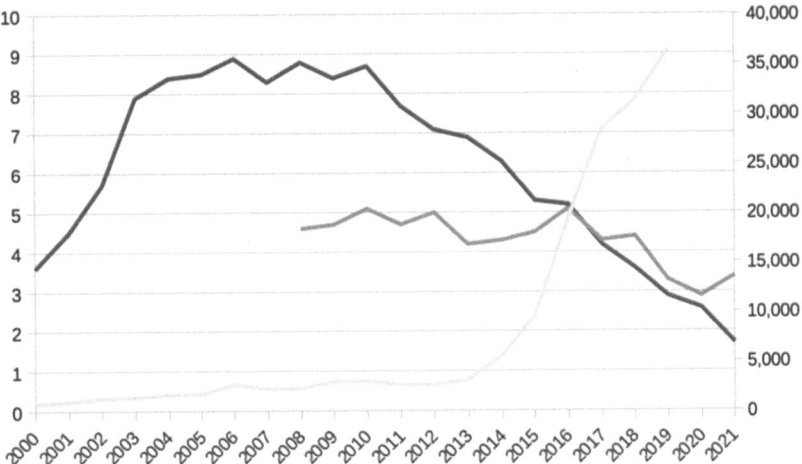

Fig. 5.1 Synthetic Opioid Use and Casualties, USA. Synthetic opioid (drugs marketed as Vicodin, OxyContin, and Percocet) use increased sharply among 19- to 30-year-olds until 2010 (12-month prevalence, blue line, left scale, in percentage). The prevalence for 35- to 59-year-olds has only been measured since 2008 (red line). The deaths related to overdoses have increased strongly since 2014 (yellow line, right scale). Note that some popular statistics include drug-related suicides, homicides, and casualties from accidents and the like, and thus report higher numbers. (Sources: Monitoring the Future (Miech et al., 2022); US National Center for Health Statistics, Data Brief 394)

problematic behaviors may remain even if the overall prevalence decreases; and, on the other hand, regulation can exacerbate existing drug-related problems. Synthetic opioids—much stronger than opium or heroin—obviously did not suddenly become more dangerous from 2014 onward, but most likely their restricted availability forced and still forces dependent users to take greater risks. Meanwhile, researchers continue to develop risk assessments for commonly used and less harmful substances, such as alcohol, cannabis, and MDMA (Ecstasy), to maximize benefits, minimize harms, and make drug policy more consistent (see, for example, Rogeberg et al., 2018; van Amsterdam et al., 2021).

One topic not addressed in much detail in the book are psychedelics, which were mentioned only cursorily in Chap. 4 as instruments to gain new experiences or insights. In recent years, the alarmist and very negative presentation of these substances in the media from approximately the 1960s to 2000 has been replaced by suspiciously high expectations about their potential to treat mental disorders, such that some researchers are already awaiting an imminent "bursting of the psychedelic hype bubble" (Yaden et al., 2022). This situation is reminiscent of the expectations about the soon-to-be discovered cognitive enhancers in the early 2000s and so many other previous hypes about psychopharmacological drugs and other neuroscientific innovations (Schleim, 2014b). While their clinical potential, as well as their capacity to create meaningful experiences for the users and a better understanding of brain function for the researchers is not denied here (see Letheby, 2022; Nutt, 2020; Vollenweider & Preller, 2020), we should also be careful not to perceive them as the next "miracle drug"—which will probably remain a mere miracle forever.

5.3   Personal Conclusion

The book will have succeeded, in my view, if it makes at least some people reconsider their views on mental health and substance use. Both of these areas of research are complex, highly dynamic, and presently receiving huge public interest. This comes with opportunities as well as risks. One risk is the continued wasting of huge amounts of funding to find a needle (i.e., identify mental disorders) in a haystack (i.e., the nervous system), when the needle probably does not even exist. One opportunity consists in finding a more consistent and generally beneficial way to deal with instrumental substance use.

In an environment in which there is much competition and performance pressure, there will always be incentives to change body and mind such that one has an advantage over others or simply copes better with stress. Acknowledging this more explicitly may be one way to address potential problems that arise from this. For example, there has been an initiative to add contextual information about how image processing is used to improve fashion models' looks in advertisements. The model Cindy Crawford once famously said that even she does not wake up looking like Cindy Crawford, indicating that she differs from the media portrayals of her. At least in highly competitive contexts, it might increase fairness and transparency to also declare one's instrumental substance use—undertaken to achieve certain aims.

In this respect, I should start out by stating that while writing this book I increased my coffee consumption from one mug after lunch to an additional mug in the morning. I also had one to two alcoholic drinks in the afternoon and evening to increase arousal and motivation, possibly also to cope with stress. Of course, I cannot tell whether the book would have been different without this substance use or whether it would just have taken longer to write. While many of my friends and acquaintances experiment with other mind-altering drugs, some of them regularly, my own further drug life is rather boring: I consumed cannabis products as a teenager, but stopped when negative experiences (in particular anxiety) became increasingly common under the influence of the substance.

My own relation with cognitive enhancement has always been ambiguous. In my final years at the *Gymnasium* (German grammar school), when I eventually enjoyed studying after a lengthy period of refusal, I experimented with high-dose caffeine tablets that could only be bought in a pharmacy. In our final yearbook, my fellow students wrote about me that: "Stephan takes caffeine instead of sleep." This was of course an exaggeration, but not without a kernel of truth. I stopped experimenting with the tablets after a couple of months, as their primary effects seemed to be increased nervousness and sweating.

Later at the university (in the early 2000s), I started reading the neuroethics literature summarized in Chap. 3. I remember giving some enthusiastic presentations on neuroenhancement at the beginning of my PhD period (starting 2005), for which I also pulled a couple of all-nighters, but then they were based on a combination of intrinsic motivation, performance pressure, and coffee. I eventually gave up my own plans to pursue a dissertation on that topic after a first review of the actual pharmacological possibilities for healthy subjects (Schleim et al., 2007; Schleim & Walter, 2007). In my view, our conclusion back then—that the expectations of what is possible with the drugs available was exaggerated—is still valid 16 years later. I then pursued research on the neuroscience of moral decision-making instead, which some also include under neuroethics (Schleim et al., 2011).

My mistake was to disregard the neuroenhancement case and consider it as "just another hype", and particularly to underestimate how long it would continue. This is what I meant by the expression that "the hype is the reality" in Chap. 3. However, the neuroethics literature available provided a welcome opportunity to address the topic in my teaching, as described in the *Frauengold* example in the preface. This allowed critical reflection on the performance society we live in, in collaboration with more than 4000 psychology students thus far, and in much more detail with small groups in the Honours College of my university. The latter students are, of course, selected for being high performers and thus generally endorse the idea of working hard to achieve something, though the majority state that they do not need substances to do so and that they can manage the stress levels.

Nonetheless, they often ask me whether I would consume substances to perform better—which I just admitted above. More answers can be found in my "Brain Doping FAQ" (Schleim, 2022a). Concerning the frequently discussed prescription stimulants, I can still say, as I did 16 years ago, that the evidence on their benefits does not look very convincing. But I still think that instrumental substance use is an important and useful concept for the future, inviting curious people to engage in theoretical research—as well as practical exploration.

Acknowledgments The idea behind the book was probably already born ten years ago, when we at the Department for Theory and History of Psychology at the University of Groningen still enjoyed lunches with our former chair in theoretical psychology, Trudy Dehue (now retired). We often talked about mental health and enhancement and found that the treatment of those with "abnormal" functioning and the enhancement of those deemed "normal" reflects two points along a continuum rather than a categorical distinction. Some of these ideas were addressed in Trudy's (Dutch) book *Better People: On Health as a Choice and a Commodity*, published in 2014. The imminent termination of the "History of Neuroethics" research project, funded by the Dutch Research Organization (NWO, grant number 451-15-042), provided a final reason to finish the book at the present time, as well as the funds to make it available for free online.

The major contribution concerning instrumental substance use came from Christian P. Müller, professor for psychiatry/addiction medicine at the University Hospital Erlangen, Germany. We met for the first time at the "Altered States" exhibition and meeting organized by the Kunstpalais in Erlangen in 2018. Over the course of at least ten years, Boris B. Quednow, professor of experimental pharmacopsychology at the University Hospital Zurich, provided major support in helping me to better understand how some of the psychoactive substances work. In spite of his busy schedule, he often replied to my questions very promptly. That we were among the few scholars who consistently doubted some of the poorly or even entirely untested hypotheses in the neuroenhancement debate led us to maintain contact for a long period and to publish a couple of articles together.

I would also like to thank Jan Christoph Bublitz, legal scholar at the University of Hamburg, and coeditor of the series in which this book is published. His feedback on the (nearly) finished book manuscript was very helpful. The participants of our monthly Theory and History of Psychology Forum at the University of Groningen, particularly Kim M. Hajek, historian at the University of Leiden, deserve my gratitude as well: We actually discussed this book project twice, first in 2021 when it was hardly more than a collection of thoughts and ideas, and then again in 2022, when it was completed. Finally, I would like to thank the Language Center of the University of Groningen for helping me to improve the manuscript.

References

Aikins, R., Zhang, X., & McCabe, S. E. (2017). Academic doping: Institutional policies regarding nonmedical use of prescription stimulants in U.S. higher education. *Journal of Academic Ethics, 15*, 229–243.

Anon. (1937). Benzedrine Sulfate 'pep pills' [editorial]. *Journal of the American Medical Association, 108*, 1973–1974.

Davis, J. E. (2020). *Chemically imbalanced: Everyday suffering, medication, and our troubled quest for self-mastery.* University of Chicago Press.

Dresler, M., Sandberg, A., Bublitz, C., Ohla, K., Trenado, C., Mroczko-Wąsowicz, A., Kühn, S., & Repantis, D. (2019). Hacking the brain: Dimensions of cognitive enhancement. *ACS Chemical Neuroscience, 10*, 1137–1148.

Duff, C. (2013). The social life of drugs. *International Journal of Drug Policy, 24*, 167–172.

Fomiatti, R., Moore, D., & Fraser, S. (2019). The improvable self: Enacting model citizenship and sociality in research on 'new recovery'. *Addiction Research & Theory, 27*, 527–538.

Foucault, M. (1978). *The history of sexuality.* Pantheon Books.

Greely, H., Sahakian, B., Harris, J., Kessler, R. C., Gazzaniga, M., Campbell, P., & Farah, M. J. (2008). Towards responsible use of cognitive-enhancing drugs by the healthy. *Nature, 456*, 702–705.

136   S. SCHLEIM

Hacking, I. (1999). *The social construction of what?* Harvard University Press.
Johnson, D. (2008). "How do you know unless you look?": Brain imaging, bio-power and practical neuroscience. *Journal of Medical Humanities, 29,* 147–161.
Letheby, C. (2022). Naturalistic entheogenics: Précis of philosophy of psychedelics. *Philosophy and the Mind Sciences, 3,* 9627.
Lewis-Fernandez, R., Rotheram-Borus, M. J., Betts, V. T., Greenman, L., Essock, S. M., Escobar, J. I., et al. (2016). Rethinking funding priorities in mental health research. *British Journal of Psychiatry, 208,* 507–509.
Malabou, C. (2008). *What should we do with our brain?* Fordham University Press.
Mazanov, J. (2019). How to respond to the increasing use of cognitive enhancers in academia? In K. van de Ven, K. Mulrooney, & J. McVeigh (Eds.), *Human enhancement drugs* (pp. 297–312). Routledge.
Meerloo, A. M. (1937). Benzedrinesulfaat als hersenstimulans. *Nederlands Tijdschrift voor Geneeskunde, 81,* 5797–5799.
Miech, R. A., Johnston, L. D., O'Malley, P. M., Bachman, J. G., Schulenberg, J. E., & Patrick, M. E. (2022). *Monitoring the Future national survey results on drug use, 1975–2021: Volume I, Secondary school students.* Institute for Social Research, The University of Michigan.
Miller, G. F. (2011). Optimal drug use and rational drug policy. *Behavioral and Brain Sciences, 34,* 318–319.
Mirowsky, J., & Ross, C. E. (2012). *Social causes of psychological distress* (2nd ed.). AldineTransaction.
Moncrieff, J., Cooper, R. E., Stockmann, T., Amendola, S., Hengartner, M. P., & Horowitz, M. A. (2022). The serotonin theory of depression: A systematic umbrella review of the evidence. *Molecular Psychiatry,* 1–14. https://doi.org/10.1038/s41380-022-01661-0
Müller, C. P. (2020). Drug instrumentalization. *Behavioural Brain Research, 390,* 112672.
Nietzsche, F. W. (1882/2006). *The Gay science.* Dover Publications.
Nutt, D. J. (2020). *Drugs—Without the Hot Air: Minimizing the harms of legal and illegal drugs* (2nd ed.). UIT Cambridge.
Quednow, B. B. (2010). Ethics of neuroenhancement: A phantom debate. *BioSocieties, 5,* 153–156.
Racine, E., Sattler, S., & Boehlen, W. (2021). Cognitive enhancement: Unanswered questions about human psychology and social behavior. *Science and Engineering Ethics, 27,* 19.
Rogeberg, O., Bergsvik, D., Phillips, L. D., van Amsterdam, J., Eastwood, N., Henderson, G., Lynskey, M., Measham, F., Ponton, R., Rolles, S., Schlag, A. K., Taylor, P., & Nutt, D. (2018). A new approach to formulating and appraising drug policy: A multi-criterion decision analysis applied to alcohol and cannabis regulation. *International Journal of Drug Policy, 56,* 144–152.

Rose, N. (2010). 'Screen and intervene': Governing risky brains. *History of the Human Sciences, 23*, 79–105.

Sahakian, B., & Morein-Zamir, S. (2007). Professor's little helper. *Nature, 450*, 1157–1159.

Schermer, M. (2008). On the argument that enhancement is "cheating". *Journal of Medical Ethics, 34*, 85–88.

Schleim, S. (2014a). Whose well-being? Common conceptions and misconceptions in the enhancement debate. *Frontiers in Systems Neuroscience, 8*, 148.

Schleim, S. (2014b). Critical neuroscience—or critical science? a perspective on the perceived normative significance of neuroscience. *Frontiers in Human Neuroscience, 8*, 336.

Schleim, S. (2020). Neuroenhancement as instrumental drug use: Putting the debate in a different frame. *Frontiers in Psychiatry, 11*, 567497.

Schleim, S. (2022a). *Pharmacological enhancement: The facts and myths about brain doping.* Theory and History of Psychology, University of Groningen.

Schleim, S. (2022b). Why mental disorders are brain disorders. And why they are not: ADHD and the challenges of heterogeneity and reification. *Frontiers in Psychiatry, 13*, 943049.

Schleim, S., & Quednow, B. B. (2018). How realistic are the scientific assumptions of the neuroenhancement debate? assessing the pharmacological optimism and neuroenhancement prevalence hypotheses. *Frontiers in Pharmacology, 9*, 3.

Schleim, S., Schnell, K., & Walter, H. (2007). Perspectives on psychopharmalogical enhancement. *Newsletter of the European Academy, 73*, 1–3.

Schleim, S., Spranger, T. M., Erk, S., & Walter, H. (2011). From moral to legal judgment: The influence of normative context in lawyers and other academics. *Social Cognitive and Affective Neuroscience, 6*, 48–57.

Schleim, S., & Walter, H. (2007). Cognitive enhancement: Fakten und Mythen. *Nervenheilkunde, 26*, 83–86.

Sperry, R. W. (1981). Changing priorities. *Annu Rev Neurosci, 4*, 1–15.

van Amsterdam, J., Nabben, T., Peters, G., van Bakkum, F., Noijen, J., & van den Brink, W. (2021). Voorstel voor rationeel MDMA-beleid. *Tijdschrift voor Psychiatrie, 63*, 665–672.

Vollenweider, F. X., & Preller, K. H. (2020). Psychedelic drugs: Neurobiology and potential for treatment of psychiatric disorders. *Nature Reviews Neuroscience, 21*, 611–624.

Wu, K. C.-C. (2011). Governing drug use through neurobiological subject construction: The sad loss of the sociocultural. *Behavioral and Brain Sciences, 34*, 327–328.

Yaden, D. B., Potash, J. B., & Griffiths, R. R. (2022). Preparing for the bursting of the psychedelic hype bubble. *JAMA Psychiatry, 79*(10), 943–944.

INDEX[1]

---

[1] Note: Page numbers followed by 'n' refer to notes.